Reeder and Felson's

Gamuts in
Cardiovascular Radiology

REEDER AND FELSON'S

GAMUTS IN CARDIOVASCULAR RADIOLOGY

COMPREHENSIVE LISTS OF RADIOGRAPHIC AND ANGIOGRAPHIC DIFFERENTIAL DIAGNOSIS

MAURICE M. REEDER

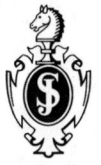

Springer-Verlag

New York Berlin Heidelberg London Paris
Tokyo Hong Kong Barcelona Budapest

Maurice M. Reeder, M.D., F.A.C.R.
Professor and Chairman, Section of Radiology, John A. Burns
    School of Medicine, University of Hawaii at Manoa,
    Honolulu, HI, USA;
Colonel, Medical Corps, United States Army, Retired;
Formerly Chief, Department of Radiology, Walter Reed Army
    Medical Center;
Formerly Radiology Consultant to the Surgeon General, United
    States Army;
Formerly Associate Radiologist, Registry of Radiologic
    Pathology, Armed Forces Institute of Pathology, Washington,
    DC, USA

Library of Congress Cataloging-in-Publication Data
Reeder, Maurice M. (Maurice Merrick), 1935–
    Reeder & Felson's gamuts in cardiovascular radiology: comprehen-
sive lists of radiographic & angiographic differential diagnosis /
Maurice M. Reeder.
        p.   cm.
    Includes bibliographical references and index.
    ISBN 0-387-94219-X (alk. paper). — ISBN 3-540-94219-X (alk.
paper)
    1. Cardiovascular system—Radiography.   2. Cardiovascular
system—Diseases—Diagnosis.   3. Diagnosis, Differential.
4. Angiography. I. Felson, Benjamin. II. Title. III. Title:
Reeder and Felson's gamuts in cardiovascular radiology. IV. Title:
Gamuts in cardiovascular radiology.
    [DNLM: 1. Cardiovascular Diseases—diagnosis.
2. Cardiovascular Diseases—radiography.   3. Diagnosis,
Differential.   4. Radiography—methods.   WG 141.5.R2 R327r
1994]
RC683.5.R3R44   1994
616.1′07572—dc20
DNLM/DLC
for Library of Congress   93-46633

Printed on acid-free paper.

Production managed by Karen Phillips; manufacturing supervised by Jacqui Ashri.
Photocomposed copy prepared from the authors' WordPerfect file using
    Ventura Publisher.
Printed and bound by Braun-Brumfield, Ann Arbor, MI.
Printed in the United States of America.

9 8 7 6 5 4 3 2 1

ISBN 0-387-94219-X Springer-Verlag New York Berlin Heidelberg
ISBN 3-540-94219-X Springer-Verlag Berlin Heidelberg New York

Dedication

This book is dedicated to Colonel William LeRoy Thompson, Medical Corps, U.S. Army (1891-1975)

Colonel Thompson, legendary teacher of morphology in radiology and originator of the Gamut concept, received his M.D. degree from the University of Pennsylvania in 1917, and began his long and illustrious career in the U.S. Army Medical Corps that same year. He had various assignments in general medicine and administration and later became one of the early Army radiologists.

It was during his last year before retirement from the Army (1951), however, that he began his most important work, his major contribution to medicine: the organization of the Registry of Radiologic Pathology at the Armed Forces Institute of Pathology. After retirement, he offered his services, without remuneration, to continue as full-time Registrar and Chief of Radiologic Pathology.

In the ensuing 16 years, Colonel Thompson worked laboriously in accessioning new material and collating the material already in the files of the Institute. He was sustained in this labor by hours of daily contact with his "students." It was here, in seminars at the viewbox, that Colonel Thompson drew upon a lifetime of accumulated knowledge and experience to educate residents, fellows, and practicing physicians from all over the world who came to study under his guidance. In this role, Colonel Thompson was the catalyst, igniting in his students a love of learning and an understanding of the vital role that pathology plays in the discipline of radiology. He was primarily a morphologist, and accepted as such by his colleagues and peers at the AFIP.

Colonel Thompson's down-to-earth nature, his éclat in interpersonal relationships, his obvious deep regard for his students as well as medicine, and his abundant and abiding warmth as a human being have made him truly beloved by all who came to know him.

A Tribute to Ben Felson

He was certainly the greatest radiologist of his time, and perhaps of all time. He was one of the great men of this century. He was also my very close and dear friend and colleague. He was like a second father to me and his loss to me is monumental, as is his loss to all whose lives he touched in such a profound and positive manner. He lived the fullest life of anyone I ever knew. He was the quintessential student and teacher, the consummate traveler, and the most compassionate, loving, and lovable human most of us have ever known.

He was that rare combination of Will Rogers and William Osler, and wherever he went, from Cincinnati to Colombia to China, he made a lasting impact and lifelong friends. More than anyone else, he enhanced the reputation and knowledge of the fledgling speciality of Radiology through his inquisitiveness and his gift for communication with both the written and spoken word. He nurtured the careers of countless students, residents, and doctors around the world. He will live forever in the hearts and minds of all who knew and loved him.

Godspeed Ben, and continue to smile down on us from above as you did so often during your all-too-brief stay with us on earth.

Maurice Reeder, M.D.

Foreword to *Gamuts in Radiology,* Third Edition

by Elias G. Theros, M.D.
I. Meschan Distinguished Professor of Radiology,
Wake Forest University Medical Center,
Winston-Salem, North Carolina, USA

Amongst the present generation of radiologists, beguiled by the glamour and excitement of the new high tech imaging and interventional modalities, too few have developed a strong sense of differential diagnosis based on radiologic pattern recognition and its correlation with clinical and laboratory findings. There is no question about the incredible contribution by the new modalities to our diagnostic armamentarium, but in the evolution of modern-day radiologic practice, the cognitive element has been neglected and our abilities as diagnosticians have suffered.

The advent of the third edition of Reeder and Felson's *Gamuts in Radiology* is timely and welcome. As always, use of the gamut lists will help evoke differential thinking, and this has been enhanced by the addition of numerous new gamuts as well as by the updating of over three-fourths of the previously existing gamuts.

Drs. Reeder and Felson in preparing these gamuts have made a major contribution to diagnosis in radiology. This they were able to do because of the depth of their own experience and their powers of observation. Those of us who have worked closely with them know that they are radiologists of consummate skills, both in the teaching and practice settings. They are master teachers to whom we all owe much. It is radiology's great fortune that Dr. Reeder has persisted, after Dr. Felson's untimely death, in laboring long hours in gamut researching and updating. He is providing his professional colleagues with an ever improving powerful diagnostic tool. We are all in his debt.

Table of Contents

Preface

The word *gamut* is defined as the whole range of any-thing. As used in this book, it indicates a complete list of causes of a particular roentgen finding or pattern.

This book, which consists of material excerpted and reorganized from *Reeder and Felson's Gamuts in Radiology, Third Edition,* was created specifically for radiologists, cardiologists, and cardiovascular surgeons. If used correct-ly, it will become an indispensable aid to pattern recognition and differential diagnosis when interpreting radiographs in the clinical setting.

Most radiologists use the "Gamut approach" without calling it that. You see an enlarged left atrium and immedi-ately search your memory bank for causes. You recall perhaps six causes, then eliminate two because of rarity or incompatible roentgen pattern. Then, with the clinical infor-mation at your elbow, you weed out two more that don't fit the clinical setting, leaving you with perhaps one or two likely diagnoses.

This process is the basis of the triangulation approach to radiologic diagnosis espoused by the originator of the gamut concept, Colonel William LeRoy Thompson. He taught that roentgen diagnosis begins with accurately interpreting all the nuances and data inherent in the radiograph, then using that information to derive a particular pattern. The second side of the triangle involves reference to a well-constructed list of differential diagnosis, which includes not only the common causes, responsible for over 80 percent of the entities, but also the uncommon causes, which are frequent-ly overlooked. The triangle is then completed by reference to the pertinent clinical and laboratory data, age, sex, and other important information concerning the patient.

The purpose of this book is to provide you with complete and accurate lists of differential diagnosis. It is an unobtru-sive consultant, quickly available whenever you interpret

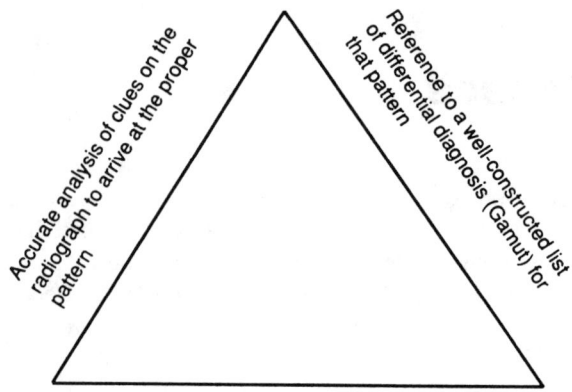

Accurate analysis of clues on the radiograph to arrive at the proper pattern

Reference to a well-constructed list of differential diagnosis (Gamut) for that pattern

Correlation of radiographic findings
and Gamut with patient's clinical
and lab findings to arrive at the
most likely diagnosis

films or prepare a presentation. In each patient, the possibilities are narrowed down to those that fit the roentgen signs and the clinical and laboratory findings. Of course, all the pertinent data on the film must be analyzed to find the appropriate roentgen sign or pattern. Study well — to identify a pattern incorrectly will land you in the wrong gamut, which could be a disaster!

Many individual gamuts that first appeared in *Gamuts in Radiology* can also be found reproduced (credited or otherwise) in a variety of publications. Many excellent texts have been published that emphasize the gamut or differential diagnosis approach, including those by Drs. Burgener and Kormano, Chen, Eisenberg, Elliott, Fraser and Pare, Sutton and Young, Swischuk, and Taybi and Lachman. However, residents and practitioners who use abbreviated lists from other, more watered-down, sources are deprived of the true worth of gamuts, which is to provide a comprehensive listing of the multiple causes, both common and uncommon, for a particular pattern. The point is to jog your memory to recall *all* the various possibilities for any given finding.

We are the first to admit that the amount of information and knowledge required to analyze with unerring accuracy and completeness all of the patterns which can present to the radiologist is beyond the comprehension of any two (or perhaps twenty) individuals. Nevertheless, our combined experience of over 75 years' practice in major medical centers in the United States as well as numerous visiting professorships throughout virtually the entire world, have given us sufficient perspective to at least attempt such a prodigious endeavor. Along the way we have been greatly aided by our close association with many outstanding radiologists who broadened our horizons and added invaluable insights in their own specialty areas.

While the individual gamuts are extensively referenced, you will note that the majority of current references refer to textbooks rather than journal articles. This is because today's general and subspecialty textbooks are much more likely to refer to the multiple causes for a given pattern than individual articles, which are usually focused on specific entities or procedures. Furthermore, exhaustive lists of references would increase the book's size enormously and undermine its primary goal, which is to provide a quick, efficient reference.

You may question whether a specific listed entity can give rise to a given pattern, or whether it is a common or uncommon member of that gamut. Although there may be some errors among the many thousands of entries, virtually all listed causes have appeared in the literature or have been seen by the authors or our colleagues. Obviously, what is common in one part of the world may be rare or unknown elsewhere. For example, Chagas' disease is a common cause of myocardiopathy in South America, but is relatively unknown elsewhere. Coronary artery disease, on the other hand, is extremely common in North America and Europe, but is relatively uncommon in the tropics. Thus, while the list of causes for a specific pattern may be quite complete within each gamut, the relative prevalence of those causes can vary widely geographically.

The legendary Colonel Thompson is well remembered by his former students and disciples for his insistence on the triangulation approach to radiographic interpretation. This clinically oriented physician taught an entire generation of radiology residents and fellows the nuances of interpretation and differential diagnosis of various roentgen patterns. In today's clinical setting, where the proliferation of new technologies is colliding with ever increasing pressures to contain costs and optimize the use of diagnostic tests (as Dr. Theros has so eloquently stated in his foreword), it is more important than ever that young radiologists and clinicians learn and apply these principles, which are summarized in these remarks by the Colonel:

"The radiograph is to the radiologist what the gross specimen is to the pathologist. It is a window on the disease, mirroring the many changes occurring within the patient during the course of an illness."

"The clues to the pattern (and often the diagnosis itself) are almost always on the film if you are observant enough and smart enough to pay attention to all the data inherent in the radiograph."

"Remember that the radiograph is only one-tenth of a second in the history of a disease process. You must always think back to what the findings looked like a day or a week or a year ago (preferably with the help of old films if available, but using intuition or deductive reasoning in their absence) and think ahead to what the findings are likely to be tomorrow or next week."

"A good radiologist must be a good anatomist and morphologist and have a clear understanding of the correlation between what is seen on the radiograph and the underlying gross and microscopic pathology."

Finally, I would like to add a few of my own thoughts that I have passed on to residents over the years.

"The radiograph is only one piece of the diagnostic puzzle. It must be evaluated in light of what you know about the patient. The radiologist cannot function as an isolated island unto himself. He or she needs a knowledge of differential diagnosis together with clinical information and interaction with the patient's physician to arrive at the proper solution."

"The radiograph is like a single page in a mystery novel. To find out 'whodunit' you usually need more detailed information than is available at a single glance."

"Remember that what comes out of the automatic processor so often is not a diagnosis but rather a diagnostic challenge, a pattern for which there may be four or forty possible causes. It is up to us, as the physician's consultant, to interpret this pattern correctly using the triangulation approach."

"With newer modalities such as MRI, it is becoming increasingly important to be conversant with the science behind the images (eg, T1 and T2 changes)."

"The ideal radiologist (or cardiologist or surgeon who routinely analyzes radiographs or angiograms) should combine exceptional visual acuity with the intuition of a good detective, the solid background of a scientist, and the knowledge of odds of a smart card player. It is these qualities and attention to detail that set him or her apart from others who merely 'look at' films."

And perhaps the most important advice to residents and young physicians: "Work hard and play hard. Enjoy your work and free time. Life is short."

MMR

Acknowledgments

In creating a project of this magnitude, the authors will inevitably borrow freely from many sources. Specific citations follow most gamuts, and a list of more general references appears at the end of this volume. For those instances where debts are not acknowledged, the reader should understand that lost notes and jaded memories, not ingratitude, are to blame.

The published works of the following outstanding radiologists resulted in valuable additions to many of the gamuts found in this book: Drs. Kurt Amplatz, Francis A. Burgener, W. R. Castañeda-Zuñiga, J. Chen, Ronald L. Eisenberg, Larry Elliott, Robert Fraser, Eugene Gedgaudas, E. Robert Heitzman, William Meszaros, A. J. Moss, Frederick Silverman, David Sutton, Leonard E. Swischuk, Hooshang Taybi, and, of course, Benjamin Felson, the renowned co-author of the two previous editions of the complete *Gamuts in Radiology* text. We want to especially thank Dr. Elias G. (Lee) Theros for his insightful foreword to this text.

The production and distribution of this book would not have been possible without the unwavering faith and guidance of the Editorial and Book Production staffs of Springer-Verlag New York, who kept the project on track to assure the timely publication of a highly refined end product.

An Appreciation

To my wife, Barbara, whose patience, love, and perseverance made possible the timely publication of this present work, and to the entire Reeder family, and to those colleagues, mentors, and friends, past and present, who have so indelibly defined my own career:

> *William LeRoy Thompson*
> *Benjamin Felson*
> *Elias G. Theros*
> *Philip E. S. Palmer*
> *Harold G. Jacobson*

> MMR

How To Use This Book

1. TABLE OF CONTENTS

This book has an extensive index. In addition, each subsection has its own table of contents. It will pay you to take a few minutes to look over the subheadings in the table of contents of each subsection. Gamuts are grouped in what we consider a logical manner. However, our logic may not be your logic; if you don't find a gamut where you think it belongs, scan the entire table of contents of that subsection or refer to the index before assuming that it is absent.

2. SUBGAMUTS

A subgamut amplifies some part of the gamut to which it belongs. Be sure to refer to it after you have finished with the parent gamut.

3. INCIDENCE

In most of the gamuts, the entities are subdivided into two groups, *Common* and *Uncommon*. These refer to the relative, rather than absolute, incidence of the disease. Although a coronary artery aneurysm (Gamut C-56) is an uncommon roentgen finding, if you do see one, the etiology will generally prove to be atherosclerosis or congenital as listed under *Common*. However, there are at least eleven other *Uncommon* entities that must be considered in the differential diagnosis.

The prevalence of many disorders varies both geographically and from one type of institution to another. To avoid major discrepancies, we have based our incidence estimates on our experience at Theoretical General Hospital, Midland, U.S.A.

Admittedly, some of the gamuts deal with seldom seen roentgen signs, but it is in just this type of situation that a gamut is most welcome. It substitutes someone else's experience for your own lack of it.

4. ALPHABETICAL LISTING

The entries in each gamut have been alphabetized for your convenience. Since the entry may not be listed in the form that first comes to your mind, be sure to scan the entire gamut before assuming that a condition is not included. Abbreviations are listed on page 129.

5. SUPPLEMENTARY GAMUTS

Most of the gamuts refer to a roentgen sign, pattern, or complex. However, interspersed throughout the book are classifications, anatomic and physiologic gamuts, and other information useful to the radiologist and clinician. A typical example is Gamut C-5A (Differential Features of Common Left to Right Shunts).

6. TERMINOLOGY

We have usually selected the most widely used terms for each disease, often furnishing a synonym or eponym as well.

In order to shorten the gamut lists, similar or related conditions are combined, often separated by a comma or semicolon (eg, PDA; aortopulmonary window). Inclusive group designations, such as lymphoma or bleeding or clotting disorders, are often utilized. In these instances you will find the subscript $_g$, which tells you to look in the Glossary (page 131) if you want to know all the entities in that group. Example: Anemia, primary$_g$. If one member of a group is a more likely cause of a particular roentgen finding, it is specifically listed. To illustrate: Anemia, primary$_g$ (esp. sickle cell).

7. BRACKETS

Brackets are used to indicate a condition that does not actually cause the gamuted roentgen finding, but can produce roentgen changes that simulate it. In Gamut C-45 (Prominence of the Main Pulmonary Artery Segment) *mediastinal or left hilar mass,* which is not a cause, but a mimic, is bracketed.

8. SYNDROMES

S. stands for Syndrome. We must apologize for the great number of congenital syndromes we have included. Since the information is available, we could hardly ignore it. Lump them together? The pediatric roentgenologists had just split them apart. We had a huge tiger by the tail, an animal with variegated stripes and swollen gamuts. Seckel's bird-headed dwarfism, VATER, and prune-belly syndromes, indeed! They should have their own Gamut Book. We can only advise those of you who seldom see dwarfs and other little people to ignore these entries. For those who are interested, it will be useful to consult Taybi and Lachman's syndrome book for definitions of these congenital disorders.

9. REFERENCES

References are used to cite only articles, books, and other contributions that have provided a number of the disease entities listed in a gamut. To document each entity would be an impossible task. A listing of general references appears in the back of the book.

10. ALTERATIONS

We are fully aware that there are omissions on the Gamut lists. Very rare entities or syndromes or single case reports have been deliberately omitted. There are also some inconsistencies in terminology, coverage, and unity. There may even be occasional factual inaccuracies. We hope these flaws are neither too frequent nor too annoying.

Please correct errors if you encounter them; delete entities that you feel do not belong on a gamut; insert additional disorders and add new gamuts as you discover them in the literature or in your practice; create some gamuts yourself. Send us your changes, with documentation, so that they can be incorporated in future editions.

C

Cardiovascular Gamuts

OTHER CARDIAC OR PERICARDIAL ABNORMALITIES

ASSOCIATED PULMONARY AND THORACIC ABNORMALITIES

Gamut C-1

CONGENITAL SYNDROMES WITH CONGENITAL HEART DISEASE

COMMON

1. Adrenogenital S., Addison's disease (aortic, tricuspid, or mitral insufficiency)
2. Asplenia S., polysplenia S. (complex cyanotic conditions)
3. Chondrodysplasia punctata (VSD, PDA)
4. Chondroectodermal dysplasia (Ellis-van Creveld S.) (septal defects, common atrium)
5. Chronic granulomatous disease of childhood (aortic stenosis)
6. Crouzon S. (PDA, coarctation)
7. Diabetic mother S. (cardiomyopathy, IHSS)
8. Down S. (VSD, ASD, AV communis)
9. Ehlers-Danlos S. (medial necrosis of aorta, dissecting aneurysm, aortic insufficiency, mitral valve prolapse)
10. Fetal alcohol S. (septal defect)
11. Friedreich's ataxia (myocardiopathy)
12. Holt-Oram S. (ASD, VSD)
13. Homocystinuria (medial degeneration of aorta and pulmonary artery causing dilatation; arterial and venous thromboses)
14. Kartagener S., immotile cilia S. (dextrocardia or situs inversus; septal defects)
15. Marfan S. (aortic or mitral insufficiency, cystic medial necrosis of aorta or occasionally pulmonary artery, dissecting aneurysm)
16. Mucopolysaccharidoses (eg, Morquio S., Maroteaux-Lamy S., Scheie S.—aortic insufficiency; Hurler S., Hunter S.—intimal thickening of coronary arteries and valves, myocardial disease)
17. Myotonic dystrophy (conduction abnormalities, mitral valve prolapse)
18. Neurofibromatosis (pulmonary stenosis, aortic stenosis, coarctation, VSD)

(continued)

19. Osteogenesis imperfecta (aortic or mitral valvular incompetence)
20. Rubella S. (PDA, VSD, PS, pulmonary artery branch stenosis)
21. Tuberous sclerosis (myocardiopathy, rhabdomyoma of heart)
22. Turner S. (coarctation of aorta, pulmonary stenosis, aortic stenosis, ASD)
23. Venolobar or scimitar S. (partial APVR)
24. Williams S. (supravalvular aortic stenosis, pulmonary artery branch stenoses)

UNCOMMON

1. Aase-Smith S. (VSD, coarctation)
2. Aminopterin fetopathy (various)
3. Apert S. (VSD)
4. Carcinoid S. (endocardial fibrosis with tricuspid valve lesions, PS)
5. Cardiofacial S. (various)
6. Carpenter S. (PDA)
7. Cerebrohepatorenal S. (PDA, septal defects)
8. Chromosomal deletion S.: 4p–; 5p– (cat cry S.); 18q– (ASD, VSD, PDA)
9. Cornelia de Lange S. (various)
10. Cutis laxa (coarctation, pulmonary artery stenoses)
11. Deaf-mutism (pulmonary stenosis, mitral insufficiency)
12. DiGeorge S. (right arch, coarctation of aorta, tetralogy)
13. Duchenne's muscular dystrophy (myocardiopathy)
14. Fanconi S. (hypoplastic left heart)
15. Fetal hydantoin S. (various)
16. Forney S. (mitral insufficiency)
17. Goldenhar S. (PDA, VSD, tetralogy, coarctation)
18. Goltz S. (aortic stenosis)
19. Gorlin S. (PDA)
20. Hallermann-Streiff S. (various)
21. Kawasaki S. (coronary artery aneurysms; pancarditis)
22. Laurence-Moon-Biedl S. (tetralogy, VSD)
23. LEOPARD S. (multiple lentigenes S.) (pulmonary stenosis, aortic stenosis)

24. Lutembacher's S. (rheumatic mitral stenosis and ASD)
25. Noonan S. (stenosis of pulmonary valve or pulmonary artery branches, ASD, VSD, myocardiopathy)
26. Pompe's disease (persistence of left supracardinal vein; myocardiopathy)
27. Prune-belly S. (PDA, VSD)
28. Radial aplasia-thrombocytopenia (TAR) S. (ASD, tetralogy, dextrocardia)
29. Refsum S. (AV conduction defect)
30. Rubinstein-Taybi S. (PDA)
31. Seckel S. (VSD, PDA)
32. Smith-Lemli-Opitz S. (VSD, PDA)
33. Sturge-Weber S. (coarctation)
34. Thoracoabdominal wall defect S. (dextrocardia, pericardial hernia, left ventricular diverticulum)
35. Treacher Collins S. (VSD, PDA, ASD)
36. Trisomy 13 S. (VSD, ASD, PDA, dextrocardia)
37. Trisomy 18 S. (VSD, PDA, PS, coarctation)
38. VATER S. (tetralogy, VSD)
39. Ventriculoradial S. (VSD)
40. Weill-Marchesani S. (PDA)
41. XXXXX S. (PDA)
42. XXY (Klinefelter S.), XXXY, XXYY, XXXYY S. (PDA, ASD)

References:

1. Elliott LP: Cardiac Imaging in Infants, Children, and Adults. Philadelphia: Lippincott, 1991, pp 111-112
2. Felson B (ed): Dwarfs and other little people. Semin Roentgenol 1973;8:260
3. Hurst JW, Logue RB, Schlant RC, et al: The Heart. (ed 3) New York: McGraw-Hill, 1974
4. Jones KL: Smith's Recognizable Patterns of Human Malformation. Philadelphia: W.B. Saunders, 1988
5. Mishkin FS: Lung curve indicating a left-to-right shunt in an infant with a large heart. Semin Nucl Med 1981;11:161-164
6. Moss AJ, Adams FH, Emmanouilides GC: Heart Disease in Infants, Children and Adolescents. (ed 2) Baltimore: Williams & Wilkins, 1977
7. O'Brien KM: Congenital Syndromes with Congenital Heart Disease. Semin Roentgenol 1985;20:104-105

(continued)

8. Taybi H, Lachman RS: Radiology of Syndromes, Metabolic Disorders, and Skeletal Dysplasias. (ed 3) Chicago: Year Book Medical Publ, 1990, p 831
9. Wilson JD, et al: Harrison's Principles of Internal Medicine. (ed 12) New York: McGraw-Hill, 1991

Gamut C-2

RELATIVE INCIDENCE OF VARIOUS CONGENITAL HEART DISEASES[*] (IN ORDER OF DECREASING FREQUENCY)

COMMON

1.	VSD	20-25%
2.	PDA	12-15%
3.	Tetralogy of Fallot$_g$	11-15%
4.	Pulmonary stenosis	10-15%
5.	ASD	7-14%
6.	Transposition of great vessels	5-9%
7.	Coarctation of aorta	5-9%
8.	Aortic stenosis	3-6%

UNCOMMON

1.	Single ventricle	2-3%
2.	Tricuspid atresia	1.2-3%
3.	Corrected transposition	1.2-3%
4.	Truncus arteriosus	1-3%
5.	AV canal defect	2%
6.	TAPVR	2%
7.	Aortic atresia	2%
8.	Pulmonary atresia	1-1.7%
9.	Endocardial fibroelastosis	1%
10.	Ebstein's anomaly	1%

[*] All others are very rare (less than 1%).

Reference:

1. Burgener FA, Kormano M: Differential Diagnosis in Conventional Radiology. (ed 2) New York: Thieme Medical Publ, 1991, p 315

Gamut C-3

KEY FINDINGS IN NEONATAL CONGENITAL HEART DISEASE

PULMONARY VASCULARITY	CONGESTIVE FAILURE Early	Late	CYANOSIS Early*	Late
I. Increased (Shunt + Pulmonary Venous Hypertension)				
COMMON				
1. Coarctation S. (coarctation + VSD and/or PDA)		+		
2. Complete atrioventricular canal		+		
3. Complete transposition of GV			+	
4. Hypoplastic left heart S_g (eg, aortic atresia with ASD and PDA)	+		+	
5. PDA—preterm infant	+			
6. Persistent fetal circulation			+	
7. TAPVR (above diaphragm)		+		
8. Truncus arteriosus		+		
9. VSD		+		
UNCOMMON				
1. ASD		+		
2. Common atrium		+		
3. Double outlet RV		+		+
4. Hemitruncus		+		
5. Peripheral AVM	+			
6. Single ventricle with transposition		+		+

(continued)

PULMONARY VASCULARITY	CONGESTIVE FAILURE Early	CONGESTIVE FAILURE Late	CYANOSIS Early*	CYANOSIS Late
II. Pulmonary Venous Hypertension (PVH)				
COMMON				
1. Aortic atresia or severe stenosis	+		+	
2. TAPVR (below diaphragm)	+		+	
UNCOMMON				
1. Anomalous origin of coronary artery from pulmonary artery		+		
2. Cardiac tumor (eg, rhabdomyoma)	+			
3. Congenital mitral stenosis	+			
4. Cor triatriatum		+		
5. Endocardial fibroelastosis		+		
6. Glycogen storage disease (Pompe-II)		+		
7. Infant of diabetic mother—myocardiopathy	+	+		
8. Myocarditis		+		
9. Pulmonary vein stenosis		+		
III. Decreased Pulmonary Vascularity				
COMMON				
1. Tetralogy of Fallot$_g$ with severe PS (incl. pseudotruncus)			+	
UNCOMMON				
1. Ebstein's anomaly			+	
2. Persistent fetal circulation			+	
3. Single ventricle with PS				+
4. Tricuspid atresia				+

* Birth to one week.

Reference: 1. Modified from Tonkin ILD: The Infant with Respiratory Distress. In: Elliott LP (ed): Cardiac Imaging in Infants, Children, and Adults. Philadelphia: Lippincott, 1991, p 777

Subgamut C-3A

NEONATAL RESPIRATORY DISTRESS

COMMON
1. Aspiration S. (eg, meconium, amniotic fluid)
2. Congenital heart disease
3. Diaphragmatic hernia
4. Hyaline membrane disease
5. Pneumonia
6. Respirator therapy (eg, PEEP); shock lung; Mikity-Wilson S.
7. Tachypnea of the newborn

UNCOMMON
1. Adenomatoid malformation of lung
2. Choanal atresia
3. Eventration or paralysis of diaphragm
4. Lymphangiectasia, congenital
5. Neuromuscular disorder$_g$ (eg, Werdnig-Hoffman S.)
6. Pierre Robin S.
7. Pulmonary edema or hemorrhage
8. Sequestration of lung
9. Tracheoesophageal fistula
10. Vascular ring

References:
1. Silverman FN (ed): Caffey's Pediatric X-ray Diagnosis. An Integrated Imaging Approach. (ed 8) Chicago: Year Book Medical Publ, 1985
2. Swischuk LE: Radiology of the Newborn, Infant, and Young Child. (ed 2) Baltimore: Williams & Wilkins, 1989
3. Wesenberg RL: The Newborn Chest. Hagerstown, MD: Harper & Row, 1973

CARDIOMEGALY OR CARDIAC FAILURE IN A NEONATE, INFANT, OR CHILD

COMMON

1. Anemia (esp. erythroblastosis, sickle cell disease)
*2. Coarctation of aorta; interrupted aortic arch
*3. Left to right shunt, large (VSD, PDA, atrioventricular canal defect)
4. Myocardiopathy (See C-32)
5. [Pericardial effusion] (See C-41)
6. Rheumatic heart disease
*7. Tetralogy of Fallot$_g$, severe (incl. pseudotruncus arteriosus)
*8. Transposition of great vessels

UNCOMMON

*1. Aortic stenosis or atresia
*2. APVR, total
3. Arrhythmia (eg, heart block, paroxysmal tachycardia)
*4. Asphyxia (esp. first day)
5. Asplenia S. or polysplenia S.
6. AV fistula or hemangioma, pulmonary or peripheral (incl. vein of Galen aneurysm, hepatic cavernous hemangioma)
7. Coronary disease (anomalous origin of left coronary from pulmonary artery; progeria; aneurysm in Kawasaki S.)
8. Cor triatriatum
9. Double outlet right ventricle
10. Ebstein's anomaly; Uhl's anomaly
*11. Endocardial fibroelastosis
*12. Fluid overload; sodium chloride poisoning
*13. Foramen ovale closure, prenatal
14. High-output state, other (eg, neonatal hyperthyroidism)
*15. Hypoplastic left heart S.$_g$

16. Increased intracranial pressure (eg, cerebral disease from birth injury)
17. Maternal diabetes, neonatal hypoglycemia
*18. Mitral stenosis or insufficiency, congenital
19. Neoplasm of heart, primary or metastatic (See C-35)
20. [Pectus excavatum; straight spine S.]
21. Polycythemia
22. [Pulmonary lymphangiectasia]
*23. Pulmonary valve atresia or severe stenosis
24. Pulmonary veno-occlusive disease (eg, atresia)
*25. Single ventricle
26. Tricuspid atresia
27. Truncus arteriosus

*Causes of congestive heart failure in first month of life.

References:

1. Elliott LP: Cardiac Imaging in Infants, Children, and Adults. Philadelphia: Lippincott, 1991
2. Moss AJ, Adams FH, Emmanouilides GC: Heart Disease in Infants, Children and Adolescents. (ed 2) Baltimore: Williams & Wilkins, 1977
3. Swischuk LE: Imaging of the Newborn, Infant and Child. Baltimore: Williams & Wilkins, 1989
4. Taybi H, Lachman RS: Radiology of Syndromes, Metabolic Disorders, and Skeletal Dysplasias. (ed 3) Chicago: Year Book Medical Publ, 1990, pp 830-831
5. Wesenberg RL: The Newborn Chest. Hagerstown, MD: Harper & Row, 1973

Gamut C-5

LEFT TO RIGHT SHUNT IN CONGENITAL HEART DISEASE

COMMON
1. ASD
2. PDA
3. VSD

(continued)

UNCOMMON

1. Aortopulmonary window
2. APVR, total or partial (incl. scimitar S.)
3. Atrioventricular canal defect
4. Coronary artery fistula to right heart or pulmonary artery (incl. anomalous origin of left coronary artery from PA)
5. Corrected transposition with VSD
6. Hemitruncus (anomalous origin of right pulmonary artery from ascending aorta)
7. Left ventricular–right atrial shunt
8. Ruptured sinus of Valsalva aneurysm into right heart
9. Sequestration of lung (eg, drainage to azygos system)
10. Tetralogy of Fallot$_g$, acyanotic ("pink")

References:

1. Edwards JE, Carey LS, Neufeld HN, et al: Congenital Heart Disease. Philadelphia: W.B. Saunders, 1965
2. Elliott LP: Cardiac Imaging in Infants, Children, and Adults. Philadelphia: Lippincott, 1991
3. Felson B (ed): Congenital heart disease, part II. Semin Roentgenol 1985;20:200
4. Ferencz C, Rubin JD, McCarter RJ, et al: Congenital heart disease: Prevalence at live birth. Am J Epidemiol 1985; 121: 31-36
5. Mishkin FS: Lung curve indicating a left-to-right shunt in an infant with a large heart. Semin Nucl Med 1981;11:161-164

Subgamut C-5A

DIFFERENTIAL FEATURES OF COMMON LEFT TO RIGHT SHUNTS

	PULM VASC	PULM ART	AORTA	SVC	LV	RV	LA	RA
1. ASD	+	+	–	–	N	+	N	+
2. PDA	+	+	+	N	+	N,+	+	N
3. VSD	+	+	N, –	N	N, +	+	+	N,+

Abbreviations:
+ = increased; – = decreased; N = Normal; PULM VASC = pulmonary vasculature; PULM ART = pulmonary artery segment

Gamut C-6

RIGHT TO LEFT SHUNT OR ADMIXTURE LESION IN CONGENITAL HEART DISEASE

COMMON

1. Left to right shunt with reversal (Eisenmenger physiology)
2. Tetralogy of Fallot$_g$
3. Transposition of great vessels
4. Truncus arteriosus

UNCOMMON

1. Anomalous systemic venous return to left atrium (eg, via left SVC)
2. APVR, total (above the diaphragm)
3. Coarctation of aorta, preductal; aortic atresia
4. Double outlet right ventricle
5. Ebstein's malformation with ASD
6. Hypoplastic right heart
7. Mitral atresia or stenosis
8. Pulmonary AV malformation
9. Pulmonary stenosis or atresia with intact ventricular septum and ASD (trilogy of Fallot)
10. Pulmonary vein atresia
11. Right pulmonary artery fistula to left atrium
12. Single atrium
13. Single ventricle
14. Tricuspid atresia

References:
1. Crupi G, Macartney FJ, Anderson RH: Persistent truncus arteriosus. Am J Cardiol 1977;40:569-578
2. Edwards JE, Carey LS, Neufeld HN, et al: Congenital Heart Disease. Philadelphia: W.B. Saunders, 1965
3. Elliott LP: Cardiac Imaging in Infants, Children, and Adults. Philadelphia: Lippincott, 1991
4. Felson B (ed): Congenital heart disease, part 1. Semin Roentgenol 1985;20:110

5. Ferencz C, Rubin JD, McCarter RJ, et al: Congenital heart disease: Prevalence at live birth. Am J Epidemiol 1985;121: 31-36
6. Lester RG: Radiological concepts in the evaluation of heart disease. Mod Concepts Cardiovasc Dis 1968;37:113-118
7. Moss AJ, Adams FH, Emmanouilides GC: Heart Disease in Infants, Children and Adolescents. (ed 2) Baltimore: Williams & Wilkins, 1977
8. Rees S: Arterial connections of the lung. Clin Radiol 1981; 32:1-15

Subgamut C-6A

DIFFERENTIAL FEATURES OF MAJOR CYANOTIC CONGENITAL HEART DISEASES

	CARDIAC SIZE	PULM VASC	AORTIC ARCH	EKG
1. Tetralogy of Fallot$_g$, incl. pseudotruncus (40%)*	N,+	–	R(25%)	RVH
2. Transposition of great vessels (15%)	+	+	L	RVH/LVH
3. Tricuspid atresia (10%)	N,+	–	L	LVH
4. Trilogy of Fallot (pulmonary atresia with ASD) (5%)	+	–	L	RVH
5. Truncus arteriosus (10%)	+	+,–	R(25%)	RVH/LVH

Abbreviations:

+ = increased; – = decreased; N = normal

*The five T's comprise approximately 80% of all cyanotic congenital heart disease.

Subgamut C-6B

ONSET OF CYANOSIS IN CONGENITAL HEART DISEASE

Marked Cyanosis at Birth or in First Week

1. Asplenia S. (Ivemark S.)
2. Double outlet right ventricle with pulmonary stenosis
3. Ebstein's anomaly
4. Hypoplastic left heart S_g (eg, aortic atresia or severe stenosis; interrupted aortic arch)
5. Persistent fetal circulation
*6. Pulmonary atresia
*7. Single ventricle with pulmonary stenosis and transposition
*8. Tetralogy of Fallot$_g$ (esp. pseudotruncus)
9. Transposition of great vessels, complete
*10. Tricuspid atresia

Mild or Intermittent Cyanosis at Birth or Soon After

1. APVR, total (below the diaphragm)
2. Atrioventricular canal defect
3. Large left to right shunt with failure
4. Truncus arteriosus

* Associated with pulmonary oligemia.

References:
1. Elliott LP: Cardiac Imaging in Infants, Children, and Adults. Philadelphia: Lippincott, 1991, pp 776-777
2. Felson B (ed): Congenital heart disease, part 1. Semin Roentgenol 1985;20:110
3. Rowe RD, Mehrizi A: The Neonate with Congenital Heart Disease. Major Problems in Clinical Pediatrics. Philadelphia: W.B. Saunders, 1968, vol 5

Gamut C-7

RIGHT TO LEFT SHUNT AT ATRIAL LEVEL

COMMON

1. APVR, total
2. ASD with pulmonary hypertension (Eisenmenger physiology)
3. Transposition of great vessels with interatrial communication
4. Tricuspid atresia

UNCOMMON

1. Ebstein's anomaly with interatrial communication
2. Hypoplasia of right ventricle, isolated
3. Normal newborn with patent foramen ovale
4. Pentalogy of Fallot
5. Pulmonary hypertension, primary, with interatrial communication
6. Pulmonary stenosis or atresia with intact ventricular septum and ASD (trilogy of Fallot)
7. Single atrium
8. Tricuspid stenosis with interatrial communication
9. Uhl's anomaly

References:

1. Elliott LP: Cardiac Imaging in Infants, Children, and Adults. Philadelphia: Lippincott, 1991
2. Felson B (ed): Congenital heart disease, part 1. Semin Roentgenol 1985:20:110
3. Meszaros WT: Cardiac Roentgenology. Springfield, IL: CC Thomas, 1969
4. Moss AJ, Adams FH, Emmanouilides GC: Heart Disease in Infants, Children and Adolescents. (ed 2) Baltimore: Williams & Wilkins, 1977
5. Swischuk LE: Plain Film Interpretation in Congenital Heart Disease. (ed 2) Baltimore: Williams & Wilkins, 1979

Gamut C-8

COMPLICATED ATRIAL LEVEL SHUNTS

I. CONVENTIONAL ASD ASSOCIATED WITH ANOTHER USUALLY INDEPENDENT ANOMALY

1. APVR, partial
2. Lutembacher's S. (rheumatic mitral valve stenosis and ASD)
3. Mitral valve regurgitation or prolapse (MVP); cleft mitral valve
4. Pulmonary stenosis (eg, trilogy of Fallot)
5. VSD

II. ATRIAL SEPTUM IS INTACT; SITE OF SHUNT IS DISTAL TO ATRIAL SEPTUM BUT MAY DRAIN INTO RA

1. Coronary artery fistula
2. Left ventricular—right atrial communication
3. Rupture of posterior aortic sinus aneurysm into RA

III. ASD IS PART OF A DEVELOPMENTAL COMPLEX

1. APVR, total
2. Complete atrioventricular canal (AV communis or total endocardial cushion defect)
3. Pentalogy of Fallot

Reference:

1. Elliott LP: Cardiac Imaging in Infants, Children, and Adults. Philadelphia: Lippincott, 1991, p 593

Gamut C-9

RIGHT TO LEFT SHUNT AT VENTRICULAR LEVEL

COMMON
1. Complete transposition of great vessels with VSD
2. Pulmonary atresia with VSD
3. Tetralogy of Fallot$_g$
4. VSD with pulmonary hypertension (Eisenmenger physiology)

UNCOMMON
1. Corrected transposition with VSD and predominant PS
2. Double outlet right ventricle
3. Single ventricle
4. Truncus arteriosus

References:
1. Elliott LP: Cardiac Imaging in Infants, Children, and Adults. Philadelphia: Lippincott, 1991
2. Felson B (ed): Congenital heart disease, part 1. Semin Roentgenol 1985;20:110
3. Meszaros WT: Cardiac Roentgenology. Springfield, IL: CC Thomas, 1969
4. Moss AJ, Adams FH, Emmanouilides GC: Heart Disease in Infants, Children and Adolescents. (ed 2) Baltimore: Williams & Wilkins, 1977

Subgamut C-9A

CARDIOVASCULAR ANOMALIES ASSOCIATED WITH VSD

VSD an Essential Part of the Anomaly

COMMON
1. Tetralogy of Fallot$_g$ (incl. pseudotruncus)

(continued)

UNCOMMON

*1. Complete atrioventricular canal (AV communis)
2. Double outlet left ventricle
3. Double outlet right ventricle
4. Pentalogy of Fallot$_g$
5. Truncus arteriosus

VSD Frequently Associated with the Anomaly

COMMON

1. ASD
2. Coarctation of aorta
3. PDA
4. Pulmonary stenosis
5. Transposition of great vessels

UNCOMMON

1. APVR
2. Chromosomal abnormality (eg, trisomy anomalies)
3. Ectopia cordis
4. Interruption of aortic arch
5. Left ventricular outflow tract obstruction
6. Prolapse of right aortic cusp with aortic insufficiency
7. Sinus of Valsalva aneurysm
8. Tricuspid atresia

* Anomalies associated with complete atrioventricular canal (CAVC) include asplenia S., Down S., PDA, single ventricle, and tetralogy of Fallot$_g$.

References:

1. Edwards JE: The pathology of ventricular septal defect. Semin Roentgenol 1966;1:2-23
2. Elliott LP: Cardiac Imaging in Infants, Children, and Adults. Philadelphia: Lippincott, 1991, pp 575-576

Gamut C-10

RIGHT TO LEFT SHUNT AT DUCTUS LEVEL

COMMON
1. Coarctation of aorta, preductal
2. PDA with pulmonary hypertension (Eisenmenger physiology)
3. Persistent fetal circulation

UNCOMMON
1. APVR, total
2. Interruption of aortic arch; aortic atresia
3. Mitral atresia; congenital mitral stenosis
4. Pulmonary vein atresia

References:
1. Elliott LP: Cardiac Imaging in Infants, Children, and Adults. Philadelphia: Lippincott, 1991
2. Meszaros WT: Cardiac Roentgenology. Springfield, IL: CC Thomas, 1969
3. Moss AJ, Adams FH, Emmanouilides GC: Heart Disease in Infants, Children and Adolescents. (ed 2) Baltimore: Williams & Wilkins, 1977

PULMONARY ARTERIAL VASCULARITY IN COMMON CONGENITAL HEART DISEASES
(See Gamuts C-12 to C-16)

INCREASED VASCULARITY WITH PROMINENT PULMONARY ARTERY SEGMENT

	Incidence
1. APVR	2%
2. ASD	11%
3. Atrioventricular canal defect	2%
4. PDA; aortopulmonary window	12%
5. VSD	22%

INCREASED VASCULARITY WITH FLAT OR CONCAVE PULMONARY ARTERY SEGMENT

*1. Complete transposition of great vessels	6%
*2. Double-outlet right ventricle	
*3. Truncus arteriosus (types I, II, and III)	3%

NORMAL VASCULARITY

1. Aortic stenosis	3%
2. Coarctation of aorta	7%
3. Corrected (L-loop) transposition of great vessels	
4. Endocardial fibroelastosis	2%
5. Pulmonary valvular stenosis	10%
6. Small left to right shunt	
7. Subaortic stenosis	

DECREASED VASCULARITY

*1. Ebstein's anomaly; Uhl's anomaly	1%
*2. Pulmonary atresia or severe stenosis with ASD, transposition, or single ventricle	
*3. Tetralogy of Fallot$_g$ (incl. pseudotruncus)	12%
*4. Tricuspid atresia or stenosis	3%
5. Tricuspid insufficiency	

*6. Trilogy of Fallot
*7. Truncus arteriosus, type IV

*Cyanotic lesions.

References:
1. Chen JTT: Essentials of Cardiac Roentgenology. Boston: Little, Brown, 1987
2. Gedgaudas E, Moller JH, Castaneda-Zuniga WR, et al: Cardiovascular Radiology. Philadelphia: W.B. Saunders, 1985
3. Lester RG: Radiological concepts in the evaluation of heart disease. Mod Concepts Cardiovasc Dis 1968;37:113-118
4. Swischuk LE: Plain Film Interpretation in Congenital Heart Disease. (ed 2) Baltimore: Williams & Wilkins, 1979

Gamut C-12

ACYANOTIC CONGENITAL HEART DISEASE WITH NORMAL PULMONARY VASCULARITY*

COMMON
1. Aortic stenosis
2. Coarctation of aorta
3. Pulmonary stenosis

UNCOMMON
*1. Aberrant origin of left coronary artery from pulmonary artery
*2. Aortic insufficiency
*3. Cor triatriatum
*4. Endocardial fibroelastosis
*5. Hypoplastic left heart S.$_g$
*6. Interruption of aortic arch
*7. Mitral insufficiency
*8. Mitral stenosis
*9. Myocardiopathy (eg, glycogen storage disease, rubella S., Noonan S., mucopolysaccharidoses$_g$)
10. Subvalvular aortic stenosis (IHSS)

* Normal pulmonary vasculature until left-sided heart failure develops in infancy.

Gamut C-13

ACYANOTIC CONGENITAL HEART DISEASE WITH INCREASED PULMONARY VASCULARITY
(See Gamut C-43)

COMMON
1. ASD
2. VSD
3. PDA

UNCOMMON
1. Aortopulmonary window
2. APVR, partial
3. Atrioventricular canal defect (AV communis or endocardial cushion defect)
4. Coronary artery fistula
5. Ruptured sinus of Valsalva aneurysm (into RV or occasionally RA)

References:
1. Chen JTT: Essentials of Cardiac Roentgenology. Boston: Little, Brown, 1987
2. Eisenberg RL: Clinical Imaging. An Atlas of Differential Diagnosis. (ed 2) Rockville, MD: Aspen Publ, 1992

Gamut C-14

EXAGGERATED INTRINSIC PULSATION OF CENTRAL PULMONARY ARTERIES ("HILAR DANCE") IN CONGENITAL HEART DISEASE

COMMON
1. ASD
2. VSD

UNCOMMON

1. Anomalous left coronary artery arising from pulmonary artery
2. Aortopulmonary window
3. APVR
4. Congenital sinus of Valsalva aneurysm with intracardiac perforation
5. Coronary artery fistula (into right heart)
6. Corrected transposition of great vessels with VSD
7. Pulmonary AV fistula
8. Pulmonary insufficiency; absent pulmonary valve
9. Transposition of great vessels
10. Truncus arteriosus

Reference:

1. Felson B: Chest Roentgenology. Philadelphia: W.B. Saunders, 1973

Gamut C-15

CYANOTIC CONGENITAL HEART DISEASE WITH INCREASED PULMONARY VASCULARITY
(See Gamut C-43)

COMMON

1. APVR, total (above diaphragm)
2. Transposition of great vessels, complete
3. Truncus arteriosus (types I, II, and III)

UNCOMMON

1. Aortic atresia
2. Atrioventricular canal defect, complete
3. Common atrium
4. Double outlet right ventricle; Taussig-Bing anomaly

(continued)

5. Left to right shunt with reversal (Eisenmenger physiology, esp. PDA, VSD)
6. Single ventricle
7. Tricuspid atresia without PS

References:
1. Chen JTT: Essentials of Cardiac Roentgenology. Boston: Little, Brown, 1987
2. Gedgaudas E, Moller JH, Castaneda-Zuniga WR, et al: Cardiovascular Radiology. Philadelphia: W.B. Saunders, 1985

Gamut C-16

CONGENITAL HEART DISEASE WITH DECREASED PULMONARY ARTERIAL VASCULARITY (USUALLY CYANOTIC)

COMMON
1. Tetralogy of Fallot$_g$ (incl. pseudotruncus)

UNCOMMON
1. Asplenia S.
2. Double outlet right ventricle with PS
3. Ebstein's anomaly with ASD
4. Persistent fetal circulation
5. Pulmonary atresia or severe stenosis (isolated anomaly or assoc. with ASD, transposition, or single ventricle)
6. Pulmonary stenosis with intact ventricular septum and ASD (trilogy of Fallot)
7. Transposition of great vessels, complete or corrected, with VSD and PS or atresia
8. Tricuspid atresia or stenosis with PS or atresia
9. Tricuspid insufficiency
10. Truncus arteriosus, type IV (rarely types II or III)
11. Uhl's anomaly (parchment RV)

References:
1. Chen JTT: Essentials of Cardiac Roentgenology. Boston: Little, Brown, 1987
2. Felson B (ed): Congenital heart disease, part I. Semin Roentgenol 1985;20:110
3. Gedgaudas E, Moller JH, Castaneda-Zuniga WR, et al: Cardiovascular Radiology. Philadelphia: W.B. Saunders, 1985
4. Lester RG: Radiological concepts in the evaluation of heart disease. Mod Concepts Cardiovasc Dis 1968;37:113-118
5. Schiebler GL, Miller RH, Gessner IH: The triad of cyanosis, decreased pulmonary vascularity and cardiomegaly. Radiol Clin North Am 1968;6:361-365
6. Wesenberg RL: The Newborn Chest. Hagerstown, MD: Harper & Row, 1973

Gamut C-17

FLAT OR CONCAVE PULMONARY ARTERY SEGMENT IN CONGENITAL HEART DISEASE

COMMON
1. Tetralogy of Fallot$_g$ (incl. pseudotruncus)
2. Transposition of great vessels

UNCOMMON
1. Asplenia S.
2. Corrected transposition (pulmonary artery medially positioned)
3. Double outlet right ventricle with PS
4. Ebstein's anomaly; Uhl's anomaly
5. Hypoplastic right heart S.
6. Pulmonary atresia with intact ventricular septum
7. Single ventricle with pulmonary valve stenosis
8. Tricuspid atresia or stenosis
9. Truncus arteriosus

(continued)

References:
1. Elliott LP: Cardiac Imaging in Infants, Children, and Adults. Philadelphia: Lippincott, 1991
2. Moss AJ, Adams FH, Emmanouilides GC: Heart Disease in Infants, Children and Adolescents. (ed 2) Baltimore: Williams & Wilkins, 1977
3. Swischuk LE: Plain Film Interpretation in Congenital Heart Disease. (ed 2) Baltimore: Williams & Wilkins, 1979

Gamut C-18

VASCULAR RING AND OTHER ANOMALIES OF THE AORTIC ARCH AND BRACHIOCEPHALIC ARTERIES

COMMON
1. Coarctation of aorta
   a. Preductal (infantile—long segment narrowing)
   b. Postductal (adult—short, discrete narrowing)
2. Double aortic arch
3. Left aortic arch with aberrant right subclavian artery (incl. aortic diverticulum)
4. Pseudocoarctation of aorta
5. Right anterior aortic arch (Type I) (mirror image branching of major arteries)
6. Right posterior aortic arch (Type II)

UNCOMMON
1. Anomalous innominate artery
2. Anomalous left common carotid artery
3. Cervical aortic arch (right or left)
4. Innominate artery compression S.
5. Left aortic arch, right ductus, and right descending aorta
6. Pulmonary sling (left pulmonary artery arising from right pulmonary artery)
7. Right aortic arch, left descending aorta

8. Right aortic arch, right descending aorta, and aberrant or isolated left subclavian artery arising from pulmonary artery (Type III arch)

References:

1. Baron RL, Gutierrez FR, Sagel SS: CT of anomalies of the mediastinal vessels. AJR 1981;137:571-576
2. Chen JTT: Essentials of Cardiac Roentgenology. Boston: Little, Brown, 1987
3. Edwards JE, Carey LS, Neufeld HN: Congenital Heart Disease: Correlation of Pathologic Anatomy and Angiocardiography. Philadelphia: W.B. Saunders, 1965
4. Felson B, Palayew MJ: The two types of right aortic arch. Radiology 1963;81:745-759
5. Salomonowitz E, Edwards JE, Hunter DW: The three types of aortic diverticula. AJR 1984;142:673-679
6. Shuford WH, Sybers RG, Weens HS: The angiographic features of double aortic arch. AJR 1972;116:125-140
7. Soulen RL, Donner RM: Advances in noninvasive evaluation of congenital anomalies of the thoracic aorta. Radiol Clin North Am 1985;23:727-736
8. Stewart JR, Kincaid OW, Edwards JE: An Atlas of Vascular Rings and Related Malformations of the Aortic Arch System. Springfield, IL: CC Thomas, 1964
9. Swischuk LE: Imaging of the Newborn, Infant and Child. Baltimore: Williams & Wilkins, 1989

Subgamut C-18A

CONGENITAL HEART DISEASE ASSOCIATED WITH ANTERIOR RIGHT AORTIC ARCH (TYPE I) (MIRROR-IMAGE BRANCHING)

1. Asplenia S. (30%-40%)*
2. Pseudotruncus arteriosus (pulmonary atresia with VSD) (40%-50%)
3. Tetralogy of Fallot$_g$ (25%); "pink" tetralogy (15%)
4. Transposition of great vessels with VSD and pulmonary stenosis (5%-10%)
5. Tricuspid atresia (5%)

(continued)

6. Truncus arteriosus (25%-35%)
7. Uncomplicated large VSD (2%)

* (%) refers to approximate percentage of all cases of that anomaly with a right aortic arch.

Reference:
1. Elliott L: Cardiac Imaging in Infants, Children, and Adults. Philadelphia: Lippincott, 1991, p 146

Subgamut C-18B

EXTRINSIC VASCULAR IMPRESSION ON THE ESOPHAGUS
(See Gamut C-18)

COMMON
1. Aberrant right subclavian artery
2. Aortic abnormality, acquired (eg, aneurysm$_g$, tortuosity)
3. Aortic knob
4. Coarctation of aorta
5. Right aortic arch (esp. posterior or type 2)

UNCOMMON
1. Anomalous innominate artery
2. Anomalous pulmonary venous return (type III)
3. Aortic diverticulum
4. AV malformation
5. Azygos or hemiazygos vein dilatation
6. Cervical aortic arch
7. Corrected transposition (medially placed pulmonary artery)
8. Double aortic arch
9. Enlarged "bronchial" artery (incl. truncus arteriosus, absent main pulmonary artery)
10. Pulmonary artery "sling" (anomalous origin of left pulmonary artery)
11. Pulmonary vein confluence draining into back of left atrium
12. Sequestration of lung (anomalous artery from aorta)

Subgamut C-18C

POSITIONAL ANOMALIES OF THE THORACIC AORTA

	ARCH	DESCENDING		SUBCLAVIAN ARTERY		AORTIC DIVERTICULUM	CONGENITAL HEART DISEASE
		L	R	N	ANOMALY		
Normal	L	+		+		0	rare
Anomalous descending A	L		+			rare	rare
RAA type I	R	rare	+	+	rare	0	com
RAA type II	R	rare	+	rare	com	com	rare
Cervical AA, L	L	rare	com	rare	com	com	rare
Cervical AA, R	R	+		+	com	rare	
Anomalous R subclavian artery	L	+			+	com	rare
Double AA	L&R	+				0	rare

Abbreviations:
N = Normal; A = Aorta, L = Left; com = common; + = Present; AA = Aortic arch; R = Right; 0 = Absent

Gamut C-19

ANOMALOUS ARTERIAL COMMUNICATION IN THE THORAX

DIRECT COMMUNICATION OF AORTA AND PULMONARY ARTERY

1. Aortopulmonary window
2. PDA
3. Postoperative shunt (eg, Blalock-Taussig, Waterston, Potts)
4. Pseudotruncus
5. Truncus arteriosus

AORTIC OR SYSTEMIC ARTERY ANOMALY

1. Fistula
   a. Aortic—left ventricular tunnel
   b. Brachiocephalic artery to systemic vein (eg, fistula from transverse cervical artery to internal jugular vein)
   c. Coronary artery fistula
   d. Postoperative aortic-cardiac fistula
   e. Ruptured sinus of Valsalva aneurysm into heart
   f. Systemic—pulmonary AV malformation (bronchial, brachiocephalic, or chest wall artery to pulmonary artery, pulmonary vein, or azygos system)
2. Anomalous origin of systemic artery
   a. Left coronary artery from pulmonary artery
   b. Subclavian artery from pulmonary artery

PULMONARY ARTERY ANOMALY

1. Fistula
   a. Pulmonary AV malformation
   b. Right pulmonary artery to left atrium fistula
2. Anomalous origin of pulmonary artery
   a. Left pulmonary artery from right pulmonary artery (pulmonary sling)

   b. Left or right pulmonary artery from descending aorta

   c. Right pulmonary artery from ascending aorta (hemitruncus)

3. Anomalous artery arising from aorta to supply a lung segment
   a. Sequestration of lung
   b. Venolobar S.

References:

1. Franken EA, Hurwitz RA: Radiological Society of North America Scientific Exhibit, 1973
2. Viamonte M Jr: Intrathoracic extracardiac shunts. Semin Roentgenol 1967;2:342-367

Gamut C-20

ANOMALOUS PULMONARY VENOUS RETURN (APVR) CONNECTIONS

TOTAL (TAPVR)[*]

1. Left vertical vein	37%
2. Coronary sinus	16%
3. Infracardiac (abdominal)	15%
4. Right SVC	14%
5. Right atrium	11%
6. Mixed	7%

PARTIAL (PAPVR)

1. SVC
2. Azygos vein
3. Right atrium
4. IVC, portal vein, hepatic vein (eg, scimitar S.)
5. Left innominate vein (via vertical vein)
6. Coronary sinus
7. Mixed

[*] 25% to 30% of patients with TAPVR may have other anomalies, such as VSD, PDA, coarctation, or interruption of the aortic arch.

(continued)

Reference:
1. Moes CAF, Freedom RM, Burrows PE: Anomalous pulmonary venous connections. Semin Roentgenol 1985;20:134-150

Gamut C-21

ABNORMAL CARDIAC POSITION; CARDIAC DISPLACEMENT

CONGENITAL
1. Absence of a pulmonary artery
2. Agenesis or hypoplasia of a lobe or lung; venolobar S.
3. Asplenia or polysplenia S.
4. Congenital absence of left pericardium
5. Dextrocardia, mirror-image type with situs inversus
6. Dextroposition; mesocardia
7. Dextroversion with situs solitus or situs indeterminate
8. Levoversion (levocardia with situs inversus)
9. Pectus excavatum

ACQUIRED
1. Atelectasis; fibrosis
2. Diaphragmatic hernia; elevation of hemidiaphragm
3. Emphysema, unilateral (esp. bullous)
4. Mass lesion (eg, neoplasm, aneurysm)
5. Pleural fluid or thickening; pneumothorax
6. Pneumonectomy
7. Scoliosis (heart shifted to concave side)
8. Technical (rotation of patient)

References:
1. Baron RL, Gutierrez FR, Sagel SS: CT of anomalies of the mediastinal vessels. AJR 1981;137:571-577
2. Cooley RN: Editorial: Congenital dextrocardia and the general radiologist. AJR 1972;116:211-214
3. Felson B: Chest Roentgenology. Philadelphia: W.B. Saunders, Co.,1973

4. Majeski JA, Upshur JK: Asplenia syndrome: A study of congenital anomalies in 16 cases. JAMA 1978;240:1508-1510
5. Stanger P, Rudolph AM, JE Edwards: Cardiac malpositions: An overview based on study of sixty-five necropsy specimens. Circulation 1977;56:159-172
6. Tonkin ILD, Tonkin AK: Visceroatrial situs abnormalities: Sonographic and computed tomographic appearance. AJR 1982;138:509-515
7. Van Praagh R: The importance of segmental situs in the diagnosis of congenital heart disease. Semin Roentgenol 1985;20:254-271

Subgamut C-21A

DEXTROCARDIA

1. **Situs inversus** (all visceral organs opposite of normal; slightly increased incidence of cardiac anomalies in 5% to 10% of patients)
2. **Dextroposition with situs solitus** (cardiac apex displaced into right hemithorax—eg, hypoplasia of right lung, venolobar S.)
3. **Dextroversion with situs solitus** (anatomic relations are normal, but cardiac apex is in right side of chest—due to abnormal rotation of embryonic cardiac loop)
4. **Dextrocardia with situs ambiguus in asplenia S.** (bilateral right-sidedness) (absent spleen, three lobes in each lung, left lobe of liver same size as right lobe, malrotation of bowel, cardiac apex in either hemithorax—cardiac anomalies include common atrium, single ventricle, PS, transposition of great vessels, and TAPVR)
5. **Dextrocardia with situs ambiguus in polysplenia S.** (bilateral left-sidedness) (each lung has two lobes, hepatic segment of IVC is absent, cardiac apex is in right hemithorax in 50% of patients—cardiac anomalies include ASD, PAPVR, and interruption of IVC with azygos continuation)

Reference:
1. Gedgaudas E, Moller JH, Castaneda-Zuniga WR, Amplatz K: Cardiovascular Radiology. Philadelphia: W.B. Saunders, 1985, pp 175-181

Gamut C-22

RIGHT ATRIAL ENLARGEMENT

COMMON

1. Left to right shunt into right atrium (eg, ASD, patent foramen ovale, atrioventricular canal defect, APVR, left ventricular–right atrial shunt, ruptured sinus of Valsalva aneurysm into right atrium)
2. [Pericardial cyst, lipoma, or encapsulated fluid]
3. Pulmonary stenosis
4. Right heart failure, any cause (See C-46)
5. Right ventricular enlargement resulting in atrial enlargement (esp. cor pulmonale, mitral stenosis, chronic left heart failure) (See C-23)
6. Tetralogy of Fallot$_g$
7. Tricuspid insufficiency (See C-22A)

UNCOMMON

1. Congenital or idiopathic right atriomegaly; atrial aneurysm
2. Coronary artery fistula to RA
3. Ebstein's anomaly; Uhl's anomaly
4. Endocardial fibroelastosis
5. Endomyocardial fibrosis
6. Hypoplastic left heart S.; aortic atresia
7. Neoplasm of right atrium or ventricle (eg, myxoma) (See C-35)
8. Post–mitral valve replacement
9. Pulmonary atresia (with tricuspid insufficiency)
10. Transposition of great vessels with interatrial communication
11. Tricuspid atresia or stenosis (incl. carcinoid S.)

References:

1. Gedgaudas E, Moller JH, Castaneda-Zuniga WR, Amplatz K: Cardiovascular Radiology. Philadelphia: W.B. Saunders, 1985
2. Meszaros WT: Cardiac Roentgenology. Springfield, IL: CC Thomas, 1969
3. Rubin SA, Hightower CW, Flicker S: Giant right atrium after mitral valve replacement: Plain film findings in 15 patients. AJR 1987; 149:257-260

Subgamut C-22A

TRICUSPID INSUFFICIENCY

COMMON
1. Pulmonary hypertension
2. Rheumatic heart disease
3. Right ventricular dilatation

UNCOMMON
1. AV canal defect
2. Bacterial endocarditis (esp. in narcotics abuser)
3. Carcinoid S.
4. Ebstein's anomaly
5. Endomyocardial fibrosis
6. Myxoma of right atrium
7. Trauma
8. Tricuspid valve prolapse

Reference:
1. Wilde P, Hartnell GG: Tricuspid insufficiency. In: Sutton D, Young JWR (eds): A Short Textbook of Clinical Imaging. London: Springer-Verlag, 1990, p 176

Gamut C-23

RIGHT VENTRICULAR ENLARGEMENT

COMMON
1. Chronic left heart failure (eg, mitral insufficiency, myocardiopathy) (See C-32)
2. Cor pulmonale; pulmonary arterial hypertension, primary or secondary (eg, COPD, interstitial fibrosis, pulmonary emboli) (See C-46)
3. Left to right shunt (esp. ASD, VSD, PDA) (See C-5)
4. Mitral stenosis, acquired

(continued)

5. Pulmonary stenosis
6. Tetralogy of Fallot$_g$ (incl. pseudotruncus arteriosus)

UNCOMMON

1. Double outlet right ventricle
2. Ebstein's anomaly; Uhl's anomaly
3. Hypoplastic left heart syndrome
4. Infarction of right ventricle
5. Neoplasm of right ventricle or left atrium (eg, myxoma) (See C-35)
6. Pulmonary atresia (with tricuspid insufficiency)
7. Pulmonary insufficiency; absent pulmonary valve
8. Pulmonary venous obstruction (eg, congenital mitral stenosis, cor triatriatum, veno-occlusive disease)
9. Transposition of great vessels
10. Tricuspid insufficiency
11. Trilogy of Fallot
12. Truncus arteriosus

References:
1. Bjornsson J, Edwards WD: Primary pulmonary hypertension: A histopathologic study of 80 cases. Mayo Clin Proc 1985;60:16-25
2. Gedgaudas E, Moller JH, Castaneda-Zuniga WR, Amplatz K: Cardiovascular Radiology. Philadelphia: W.B. Saunders, 1985
3. Holmes JC, Fowler NO, Kaplan S: Pulmonary valvular insufficiency. Am J Med 1968;44:851-862
4. Meszaros WT: Cardiac Roentgenology. Springfield, IL: CC Thomas, 1969

Subgamut C-23A

FILLING DEFECT IN RIGHT VENTRICLE ON ANGIOCARDIOGRAPHY

COMMON

1. Jet of unopacified blood (eg, VSD with left to right shunt)
2. Thrombus

UNCOMMON
1. Aneurysm or diverticulum of ventricular septum
2. Anomalous muscle bundle
3. [Bernheim S. (left ventricular hypertrophy encroaching on right ventricle)]
4. Endocardial fibroelastosis (with bulging ventricular septum)
5. Foreign body (eg, catheter)
6. Idiopathic myocardial hypertrophy (eg, IHSS)
7. Neoplasm of heart, primary or metastatic (See C-35)
8. Prolapsed valve

Gamut C-24

LEFT ATRIAL ENLARGEMENT

COMMON
1. Left ventricular failure
2. Mitral insufficiency (See C-25)
3. Mitral stenosis, congenital or acquired (incl. prolapsed mitral valve)
4. Myocardiopathy (See C-32)
5. PDA; aortopulmonary window
6. VSD

UNCOMMON
1. ASD with late reversal of shunt (Eisenmenger physiology)
2. Atriomegaly, left, congenital or idiopathic
3. Constrictive pericarditis (See C-40)
4. Coronary artery fistula
5. Double outlet right ventricle
6. Endocardial fibroelastosis
7. Mitral anulus anomaly
8. Neoplasm of left atrium (eg, myxoma) (See C-35)
9. Papillary muscle rupture

(continued)

10. Parachute mitral valve complex
11. Single ventricle (cor triloculare biatriatum)
12. Thrombus in left atrium (esp. ball-valve)
13. Transposition of great vessels
14. Tricuspid atresia
15. Trilogy of Fallot
16. Truncus arteriosus

References:
1. Burgener FA, Kormano M: Differential Diagnosis in Conventional Radiology. New York: Thieme Medical Publ, 1991, pp 324-328
2. Fowler NO: Cardiac Diagnosis and Treatment. (ed 3) Hagerstown, MD: Harper & Row, 1980
3. Gedgaudas E, Moller JH, Castaneda-Zuniga WR, Amplatz K: Cardiovascular Radiology. Philadelphia: W.B. Saunders, 1985
4. Waller BF: Nonrheumatic causes of pure mitral regurgitation. Practical Card 1985;11:69-84

Gamut C-25

MITRAL INSUFFICIENCY

COMMON
1. Bacterial endocarditis
2. Functional—left ventricular dilatation (eg, cardiac failure, coarctation of aorta, aortic insufficiency, myocardiopathy) (See C-32)
3. Mitral valve prolapse
4. Papillary muscle rupture or dysfunction (eg, infarction, ischemia, trauma)
5. Postoperative (eg, mitral valve repair, valvotomy, balloon valvoplasty; dysfunctional prosthetic mitral valve)
6. Rheumatic endocarditis
7. Ruptured chordae tendineae

UNCOMMON
1. Atrioventricular canal defect
2. Congenital valvular insufficiency

3. Corrected transposition (with anomalous left atrio-ventricular valve)
4. Ehlers-Danlos S.
5. Endocardial fibroelastosis
6. IHSS
7. Marfan S.
8. Mitral anulus anomaly or calcification
9. Neoplasm (eg, carcinoid, left atrial myxoma) (See C-35)
10. Polychondritis; osteogenesis imperfecta
11. Takayasu S.

References:

1. Elliott LP: Cardiac Imaging in Infants, Children, and Adults. Philadelphia: Lippincott, 1991, pp 531-541
2. Meszaros WT: Cardiac Roentgenology. Springfield, IL: CC Thomas, 1969
3. Sutton D, Young JWR: A Short Textbook of Clinical Imaging. London: Springer-Verlag, 1990, p 168
4. Waller BF: Nonrheumatic causes of pure mitral regurgitation. Practical Card 1985;11:69-84

Gamut C-26

EXTRA BUMP ALONG THE UPPER LEFT HEART BORDER (THE THIRD MOGUL)

COMMON
1. Aneurysm of left ventricle
2. Left atrial appendage enlargement (esp. rheumatic or congenital heart disease)
3. [Pericardial adhesion, postoperative (eg, CABG) or other]
4. [Thymus gland; mediastinal mass, esp. thymoma, thymic cyst, teratoid lesion, lymphoma$_g$]

UNCOMMON
1. Absence of the left pericardium
2. Coronary artery aneurysm; coronary AV fistula

(continued)

3. Corrected transposition or single ventricle with left-sided ascending aorta
4. Cyst (eg, pericardial; hydatid)
5. Ebstein's anomaly
6. Myocardiopathy (See C-32)
7. Neoplasm of heart or pericardium (See C-35)
8. [Pleural plaque (asbestosis)]
9. Postoperative deformity (eg, conduit, aneurysm)
10. Right atrial appendage, levoposition
11. Sinus of Valsalva aneurysm (left)
12. Tetralogy of Fallot$_g$
13. Transposition of great vessels

References:

1. Daves M: Skiagraphing the mediastinal moguls. New Physician Jan 1970, p 49
2. Swischuk LE: Plain Film Interpretation in Congenital Heart Disease. (ed 2) Baltimore: Williams & Wilkins, 1979

Gamut C-27

LEFT VENTRICULAR ENLARGEMENT

COMMON

1. Aortic insufficiency (See C-28)
2. Aortic stenosis (rheumatic; congenital—bicuspid aortic valve; degenerative—idiopathic calcific stenosis)
3. Athlete's heart (no disease)
4. Coarctation of aorta
5. Combined aortic insufficiency and stenosis (usually due to rheumatic heart disease)
6. Congestive heart failure (See C-4, C-51)
7. Coronary or arteriosclerotic heart disease (incl. myocardial infarction, left ventricular aneurysm)
8. High output heart disease (eg, anemia, AV fistula, hyperthyroidism) (See C-31)
9. Hypertension

10. Mitral insufficiency
11. Myocardiopathy, myocarditis (See C-32)
12. PDA; aortopulmonary window
13. VSD

UNCOMMON

1. Atrioventricular canal defect
2. Double outlet right ventricle
3. Endocardial fibroelastosis
4. IHSS (subvalvular aortic stenosis)
5. Neoplasm of left ventricle (See C-35)
6. [Pericardial defect, total or partial]
7. Pulmonary atresia with intact ventricular septum
8. Supravalvular aortic stenosis (eg, Williams S.)
9. Transposition of great vessels
10. Tricuspid atresia or stenosis
11. Truncus arteriosus

References:
1. Burgener FA, Kormano M: Differential Diagnosis in Conventional Radiology. (ed 2) New York: Thieme Medical Publ, 1991, pp 316-323
2. Gedgaudas E, Moller JH, Castaneda-Zuniga WR, Amplatz K: Cardiovascular Radiology. Philadelphia: W.B. Saunders, 1985
3. Meszaros WT: Cardiac Roentgenology. Springfield, IL: CC Thomas, 1969
4. Miller DH, Borer JS: The cardiomyopathies: A pathophysiologic approach to therapeutic management. Arch Intern Med 1983;143:2157-2162
5. Subramanian R, Olson LJ, Edwards WD: Surgical pathology of pure aortic stenosis: A study of 374 cases. Mayo Clin Proc 1984;59:683-690

Subgamut C-27A

RADIOLOGIC FINDINGS (PULMONARY VASCULATURE AND LV SIZE) IN COMMON DISEASES WITH LEFT VENTRICULAR STRAIN

PULMONARY VASCULATURE	SIZE OF LEFT VENTRICLE	
	Normal to Slightly Enlarged	Moderately to Markedly Enlarged
Normal	Aortic or subaortic stenosis	Aortic insufficiency
	Coarctation of aorta	Myocardiopathy
	Hypertension	Hypertension (severe)
	Athlete's heart	Pericardial effusion
Venous Congestion	Acute myocardial infarction	Congestive heart failure
		Mitral insufficiency
	Mitral stenosis	
	Hypervolemia	
	Constrictive pericarditis	
Arterial and Venous Distention	VSD (small shunt)	VSD (large shunt)
	PDA (small shunt)	PDA (large shunt)
	AV malformations	

Reference:

1. Burgener FA, Kormano M: Differential Diagnosis in Conventional Radiology. Philadelphia: W.B. Saunders, 1985, p 315 (modified)

AORTIC INSUFFICIENCY

COMMON
1. Aortic root dilatation with stretched valve ring (eg, aortic ectasia; aneurysm of ascending aorta; atherosclerosis; hypertension)
2. Atherosclerotic aortic valvulitis
*3. Medial degeneration or dissection of aorta (eg, Marfan S.) (See C-55A)
4. Rheumatic aortic valvulitis

UNCOMMON
1. Aneurysm of left ventricle, subvalvular
2. Aortic–left ventricle tunnel
3. Aortic valve stenosis
4. Aortitis (eg, syphilitic, Takayasu S., rheumatic, rheumatoid arthritis, ankylosing spondylitis, Reiter S., giant cell idiopathic)
*5. Bacterial endocarditis
6. Behcet S.
7. Blunt chest trauma
8. Collagen disease$_g$
9. Congenital valvular deformity (eg, bicuspid or fenestrated aortic valve)
10. Mucopolysaccharidoses$_g$
11. Myxomatous aortic valve degeneration
12. Postoperative (eg, after valvotomy for aortic stenosis or balloon valvoplasty)
13. Prosthetic aortic valve dysfunction, degeneration, or thrombosis
*14. Rupture of aortic cusp, traumatic or other
15. Sinus of Valsalva aneurysm, congenital or acquired (eg, syphilitic, dissecting, traumatic, mycotic, atherosclerotic)
16. Supravalvular aortic stenosis (eg, Williams S.)
17. VSD high in septum with prolapsed noncoronary aortic cusp

*Acute aortic insufficiency.

(continued)

References:

1. Fowler NO: Cardiac Diagnosis and Treatment. (ed 3) Hagerstown, MD: Harper & Row, 1980
2. Meszaros WT: Cardiac Roentgenology. Springfield, IL: CC Thomas, 1969
3. Olson LJ, Subramanian R, Edwards WD: Surgical pathology of pure aortic insufficiency: A study of 225 cases. Mayo Clin Proc 1984;59:835-841
4. Subramanian R, Olson LJ, Edwards WD: Surgical pathology of combined aortic stenosis and insufficiency: A study of 213 cases. Mayo Clin Proc 1985;60:247-254

Subgamut C-28A

PROSTHETIC VALVE REGURGITATION[*]

1. Change in size of occluding ball or disc
2. Degeneration of xenograft or homograft
3. Infection
4. Strut fracture
5. Suture line dehiscence
6. Thrombosis of prosthesis

[*] Best evaluated by 2-D echocardiography, pulsed or color flow Doppler, isotope ventriculography, or MRI.

Reference:

1. Wilde P, Hartnell GG: Prosthetic valves. In: Sutton D, Young JWR (eds): A Short Textbook of Clinical Imaging. London: Springer-Verlag, 1990, pp 220-221

HYPERTENSION AND HYPERTENSIVE CARDIOVASCULAR DISEASE

I. ESSENTIAL HYPERTENSION

II. RENAL DISEASE
1. Agenesis or hypoplasia
2. Glomerulonephritis
3. Polycystic kidneys
4. Pyelonephritis, chronic

III. RENOVASCULAR DISEASE
1. Fibromuscular hyperplasia
2. Perirenal hematoma (Page kidney)
3. Renal artery stenosis

IV. ADRENAL DISEASE
1. Adrenocortical adenoma
2. Adrenogenital S.
3. Aldosteronism
4. Carcinoma
5. Cushing S.
6. Pheochromocytoma

V. CENTRAL NERVOUS SYSTEM DISORDER
1. Familial dysautonomia (Riley-Day S.)
2. Pituitary disease (eg, Cushing S.)

VI. COARCTATION OF AORTA

VII. COLLAGEN DISEASE$_g$ (esp. lupus erythematosus, polyarteritis nodosa)

VIII. HYPERTHYROIDISM

(continued)

IX. DRUG THERAPY (eg, estrogen-containing oral contraceptives)

X. NEUROGENIC (eg, psychogenic; familial dysautonomia—Riley-Day S.)

Reference:
1. Streiter ML: Gamut: Unilateral renal lesion that may result in hypertension. Semin Roetgenol 1981;16:75-76

Subgamut C-29A

UNILATERAL RENAL LESION THAT MAY CAUSE HYPERTENSION

LESION OF RENAL ARTERY OR ITS BRANCHES
1. Aneurysm
2. Arteriolar nephrosclerosis
3. Arteritis (eg, syphilis, polyarteritis nodosa, Takayasu S., thromboangiitis obliterans, rubella S., idiopathic)
4. Atherosclerosis
5. AV malformation
6. Congenital narrowing
7. Dissection
8. Fibromuscular hyperplasia
9. Neurofibromatosis
10. Perivascular fibrosis
11. Thrombosis or embolism
12. Trauma

RENAL PARENCHYMAL DISEASE
1. Neoplasm (eg, carcinoma, sarcoma, Wilms' tumor, metastasis)
2. Obstructive uropathy
3. Ptosis of kidney
4. Pyelonephritis
5. Radiation nephritis

RENAL VEIN THROMBOEMBOLISM

RENAL COMPRESSION (PAGE KIDNEY)
1. Extrarenal mass (eg, aortic aneurysm$_g$, retroperitoneal hematoma or neoplasm, peripelvic cyst)
2. Subcapsular hemorrhage

References:
1. Bookstein JJ: Cooperative study of radiologic aspects of reno-vascular hypertension. JAMA 1977;237:1706-1709
2. Hanenson IB, Gaffney TE: Clinical recognition of renal hypertension. Semin Roentgenol 1967;2:115-125
3. Johnsrude IS, Jackson DC: A Practical Approach to Angiography. Boston: Little, Brown, 1979, pp 167-185

Gamut C-30

ISCHEMIC HEART DISEASE

COMMON
1. Coronary atherosclerosis
2. Coronary embolism or thrombosis
3. Coronary spasm

UNCOMMON
1. Anemia$_g$
2. Aortic valve stenosis; other left ventricular outflow obstruction
3. Compression of coronary arteries by neoplasm, major vessel, or muscle bridge
4. Coronary artery fistula
5. Kawasaki's disease
6. Syphilis
7. Vasculitis (eg, polyarteritis nodosa)

Reference:
1. Wilde P, Hartnell GG: Ischemic heart disease. In: Sutton D, Young JWR (eds): A Short Textbook of Clinical Imaging. London: Springer-Verlag, 1990, p 158

Subgamut C-30A

COMPLICATIONS OF MYOCARDIAL INFARCTION REQUIRING RADIOLOGICAL EVALUATION

1. Congestive heart failure
2. Left ventricular aneurysm
3. Pericardial effusion
4. Ruptured interventricular septum
5. Ruptured papillary muscle

Reference:

1. Wilde P, Hartnell GG: Ischemic heart disease. In: Sutton D, Young JWR (eds): A Short Textbook of Clinical Imaging. London: Springer-Verlag, 1990, pp 161-163

Gamut C-31

HIGH OUTPUT HEART DISEASE*

COMMON

1. Anemia (eg, sickle cell disease, thalassemia); leukemia
2. Hypervolemia (fluid overload; overtransfusion)
3. Pregnancy
4. Thyrotoxicosis

UNCOMMON

1. Athletes, highly trained
2. AV fistula or malformation, peripheral, abdominal (eg, cavernous hemangioma of liver), cerebral (eg, vein of Galen aneurysm), or pulmonary
3. Beriberi (vitamin B_1 deficiency)
4. Liver disease (eg, acute liver failure; advanced cirrhosis)
5. Obesity (Pickwickian S.)
6. Paget's disease
7. Polycythemia vera
8. Pyrexia; septic shock

* Also referred to as high-flow syndromes or hyperkinetic circulatory states.

References:
1. Elliott LP: Cardiac Imaging in Infants, Children, and Adults. Philadelphia: Lippincott, 1991, pp 563-564
2. Teplick JG, Haskin ME: Roentgenologic Diagnosis. (ed 3) Philadelphia: W.B. Saunders Co, 1976
3. Wilson JD, et al: Harrison's Principles of Internal Medicine. (ed 12) New York: McGraw-Hill, 1991

Gamut C-32

MYOCARDIOPATHY

COMMON
1. Amyloidosis
2. Collagen disease$_g$ (esp. scleroderma, lupus erythematosus, dermatomyositis, rheumatoid arthritis)
*3. Endocardial fibroelastosis
*4. Hypertrophic cardiomyopathy, primary or secondary (eg, aortic stenosis, IHSS, coarctation of aorta, hypertension)
5. Idiopathic dilated cardiomyopathy
*6. Infectious myocarditis (rheumatic fever, sepsis, diphtheria, Chagas' disease, toxoplasmosis, Coxsackie, rubella, other viral disease)
*7. Ischemia (incl. coronary disease, hypoxia)
*8. Nutritional deficiency (eg, beriberi, alcoholism, cirrhosis, starvation)
9. Thyrotoxicosis

UNCOMMON
1. Acromegaly
2. Anemia
*3. Anomalous origin of left coronary artery from pulmonary artery
4. Congenital syndromes (eg, glycogen storage disease, Hurler S.) (See C-32A)
*5. Coronary artery calcification in infants

(continued)

6. Cushing S.
7. Endomyocardial fibrosis (eg, African myocardiopathy)
8. Familial
9. Hemochromatosis
*10. Leukemia, lymphoma$_g$
11. Myxedema
*12. Neoplasm, metastatic or primary (eg, fibroma, rhab-domyoma—esp. with tuberous sclerosis) (See C-35)
13. Neuromuscular disorder (eg, Friedreich's ataxia, Duchenne's progressive muscular dystrophy)
14. Postpartum
*15. Potassium or magnesium depletion
16. Pseudoxanthoma elasticum
17. Radiation therapy
18. Sarcoidosis
*19. Subvalvular left ventricular aneurysm (African)
*20. Toxicity (eg, drugs, esp. cytotoxic, Adriamycin; chemicals; cobalt–beer drinker's heart)
*21. Uremia

*Seen in infants or young children.

References:

1. Elliott LP: Cardiac Imaging in Infants, Children, and Adults. Philadelphia: Lippincott, 1991, pp 461-481
2. Goodwin JF: Clarification of the cardiomyopathies. Mod Concepts Cardiovasc Dis 1972;41:41-46
3. Gotsman MS, van der Horst RL, Winship WS: The chest radiograph in primary myocardial disease. Radiology 1971; 99:1-13
4. Meszaros WT: Cardiac Roentgenology. Springfield, IL: CC Thomas, 1969
5. Miller DH, Borer JS: The cardiomyopathies: A pathophysiologic approach to therapeutic management. Arch Intern Med 1983;143:2157-2162
6. Perloff JK: Cardiomyopathy associated with heredofamilial neuromyopathic diseases. Mod Concepts Cardiovasc Dis 1971; 40:23-26
7. Reeder MM, Palmer PES: The Radiology of Tropical Disease. Baltimore: Williams & Wilkins, 1981
8. Rowe RD, Mehrizi A: The Neonate with Congenital Heart Disease. Major Problems in Clinical Pediatrics. Philadelphia: W.B. Saunders, 1968, vol 5
9. Wilson JD, et al: Harrison's Principles of Internal Medicine. (ed 12) New York: McGraw-Hill, 1991

Subgamut C-32A

CONGENITAL SYNDROMES WITH MYOCARDIOPATHY

COMMON
1. Gaucher's disease; Niemann-Pick disease
2. Glycogen storage disease (types II and III, Pompe's disease)
3. Hemochromatosis
4. Mucolipidoses, types II and III
5. Mucopolysaccharidoses$_g$ (esp. Hurler S.)
6. Neuromuscular disorder (eg, Friedreich's ataxia, Duchenne's muscular dystrophy, Werdnig-Hoffmann disease, Kugelberg-Welander S.)
7. Noonan S.
8. Rubella S.

UNCOMMON
1. Degos S.
2. Fabry disease
3. GM$_1$ gangliosidosis; fucosidosis; mannosidosis
4. Hyperphosphatasia
5. LEOPARD S.
6. Polymyositis, dermatomyositis
7. Pseudoxanthoma elasticum

Reference:
1. Taybi H, Lachman RS: Radiology of Syndromes, Metabolic Disorders, and Skeletal Dysplasias, (ed 3) Chicago: Year Book Medical Publ 1990, p 831

Gamut C-33

GROSSLY ENLARGED HEART

COMMON
1. Aortic insufficiency
2. Combined valvular disease (esp. mitral and aortic)
3. Congestive heart failure, advanced
4. Large left to right shunt (esp. ASD, VSD, PDA)
5. Mitral insufficiency
6. Myocardiopathy (See C-32)
7. Pericardial effusion; hemopericardium

UNCOMMON
1. Complete atrioventricular canal
2. Congenital valvular atresia
3. Ebstein's anomaly

Gamut C-34

SMALL HEART

COMMON
1. Asthenia
2. Cor pulmonale (AP view)
3. [Emphysema (eg, asthma, cystic fibrosis)]
4. Normal
5. Senile atrophy
6. Wasting disease, cachexia (eg, malnutrition, de-
   hydration, kwashiorkor, tuberculosis, cancer,
   lymphoma$_g$, anorexia nervosa, scleroderma)

UNCOMMON
1. Adrenal insufficiency (Addison's disease)
2. Adrenogenital S.
3. Blood loss, severe
4. Constrictive pericarditis (See C-40)
5. Hypovolemia (eg, burn, dysentery)

Reference:
1. Swischuk LE: Microcardia: An uncommon diagnostic problem. AJR 1968;103:115-118

Gamut C-35

CARDIAC OR PERICARDIAL NEOPLASM OR CYST

COMMON
1. Invasive pulmonary or mediastinal neoplasm (eg, from lymphoma_g, bronchogenic or esophageal carcinoma, thymoma)
2. Metastasis (eg, from lung, breast, melanoma, lymphoma_g, leukemia)
*3. Myxoma (esp. left atrial)
4. Pericardial cyst
5. Rhabdomyoma (esp. with tuberous sclerosis)
6. Sarcoma (eg, rhabdomyosarcoma, fibrosarcoma, liposarcoma, hemangiosarcoma, myxosarcoma, undifferentiated sarcoma)

UNCOMMON
1. Angioma (eg, hemangioma, lymphangioma)
2. Bronchogenic cyst (intrapericardial)
3. Chondroma; osteoma
*4. Fibroma (fibrous hamartoma)
5. Hydatid cyst
6. Lipoma
*7. Mesenchymoma, benign or malignant; leiomyoma
8. Mesothelioma
9. Papilloma
10. Pericardial diverticulum
11. Pheochromocytoma
12. Teratoma (intrapericardial)

* May show calcification in tumor.

(continued)

References:
1. Bogren HG, DeMaria AN, Mason DT: Imaging procedures in the detection of cardiac tumors with emphasis on echo-cardiography: A review. Cardiovasc Intervent Radiol 1980; 3:107-125
2. David GD, Kincaid OW, Hallerman FJ: Roentgen aspects of cardiac tumors. Semin Roentgenol 1969;4:384-394
3. Elliott LP: Cardiac Imaging in Infants, Children, and Adults. Philadelphia: Lippincott, 1991, pp 482-502
4. Gross BH, Glazer GM, Francis IR: CT of intracardiac and intrapericardial masses. AJR 1983;140:903-907
5. Klatte EC, Yune HY: Diagnosis and treatment of pericardial cysts. Radiology 1972;104:541-544
6. McConnell TH: Bony and cartilaginous tumors of the heart and great vessels. Report of an osteosarcoma of the pulmonary artery. Cancer 1970;25:611-617
7. Pinet F, Moderator: Cardiac Tumour Symposium. Ann Radiol 1978;21:315-341
8. Prichard RW: Tumors of the heart: Review of the subject and report of one hundred and fifty cases. Arch Pathol 1951;51:98-128
9. Tsuchiya F, Kohno A, Saitoh R, et al: CT findings of atrial myxoma. Radiology 1984;151:139-143
10. Wilde P, Hartnell GG: Cardiac tumors; Pericardial tumors. In: Sutton D, Young JWR (eds): A Short Textbook of Clinical Imaging. London: Springer-Verlag, 1990, pp 217-218, 229-230

Gamut C-36

CALCIFICATION IN THE HEART OR GREAT VESSELS

COMMON

*1. Aneurysm$_g$ of aorta or sinus of Valsalva (See C-55)
*2. Aortic anulus (atherosclerosis, aging, syphilis) or valve (rheumatic aortic stenosis, infective endocarditis, bicuspid aortic valve)
3. Aortitis (eg, syphilis, Takayasu S.)
4. Atherosclerosis of aorta
*5. Coronary arteriosclerosis; Mönckeberg's medial sclerosis (incl. progeria)

6. Mitral anulus (atherosclerosis, Marfan S.) or valve (rheumatic mitral stenosis)
*7. Myocardial infarction; myocardial aneurysm
*8. [Pericardial calcification, constrictive pericarditis (See C-37, C-40)]

UNCOMMON

1. Alkaptonuria (ochronosis)
2. Aneurysm of left ventricle, subvalvular (African)
*3. Coronary artery aneurysm (eg, Kawasaki S.) (See C-56)
4. Diabetes
*5. Ductus arteriosus or ligamentum
*6. Endocardial fibroelastosis
7. Endocardium (eg, jet site from ASD or VSD)
*8. Hydatid cyst
*9. Idiopathic
10. Left atrial wall (rheumatic endocarditis, severe mitral valve disease)
*11. Metastatic calcinosis (eg, hyperparathyroidism, hypervitaminosis D)
*12. Myocardiopathy (eg, IHSS, Hurler S.)
*13. Neoplasm of heart (esp. myxoma, fibroma) (See C-35)
14. Oxalosis
15. Postmyocarditis (esp. rheumatic fever)
16. Pulmonary hypertension
*17. Singleton-Merten S.
18. Thromboembolus in heart chamber (esp. with myocardial infarct or aneurysm) or in great vessel (eg, aorta, inferior vena cava, pulmonary artery)
*19. Trauma, external or iatrogenic (eg, incision, coronary bypass graft, conduit)

*May occur in children.

References:

1. Arndt RD, Smith LE, Po J, et al: Myocardial calcification of the infant heart following infarction. AJR 1974;122:133-136
2. Bisset GS III: Gamut: Cardiac and great vessel calcifications in childhood: Semin Roentgenol 1985;20:194-195
3. Kleiner JP, Way GL, Hamaker WR: Intracardiac calcification in a child. Chest 1977;72:517-518

(continued)

4. Littleton JT, Cady JB: Free-floating calculi in the pericardial cavity. AJR 1978;131:901-903
5. MacGregor JH, Chen JTT, Chiles C, et al: The radiographic distinction between pericardial and myocardial calcifications. AJR 1987;148:675-677
6. Meszaros WT: Cardiac Roentgenology. Springfield, IL: CC Thomas, 1969, p 8
7. Shabetai R: The Pericardium. New York: Grune & Stratton, 1981
8. Shapiro JH, Jacobson HG, Rubinstein BM, et al: Calcifications of the Heart. Springfield, IL: CC Thomas, 1963
9. Shawdon HH, Dinsmore RE: Pericardial calcification: Radiological features and clinical significance in twenty-six patients. Clin Radiol 1967;18:205-214
10. Teplick JG, Haskin ME: Roentgenologic Diagnosis. (ed 3) Philadelphia: W.B. Saunders, 1976

Gamut C-37

PERICARDIAL CALCIFICATION

COMMON
1. Idiopathic pericarditis
2. Purulent pericarditis
3. Tuberculosis

UNCOMMON
1. Asbestos plaques along pericardium
2. Hemopericardium
3. Rheumatic fever

References:
1. Elliott LP: Cardiac Imaging in Infants, Children, and Adults. Philadelphia: Lippincott, 1991, pp 377-378, 409
2. Roberts WC, Spray TL: Pericardial heart disease: A study of its causes, consequences, and morphologic features. Cardiovasc Clin 1976;7:11-65

Gamut C-38

GAS EMBOLISM IN THE HEART OR BLOOD VESSELS
(See Gamut C-39)

COMMON
1. Fetal death
2. Hyaline membrane disease
3. Intravascular catheterization, cannulation, or therapy (eg, umbilical vein, central venous pressure line, blood transfusion or other infusion, angiography)
4. Postoperative or intraoperative (eg, cardiac bypass, lung resection, biopsy, abdominal aortic graft)
5. Respirator therapy (eg, PEEP)
6. Resuscitation maneuver
7. Trauma, penetrating (eg, laceration, blast, percutaneous high pressure injection, air hose injection)

UNCOMMON
1. Abortion, parturition, vaginal insufflation (eg, cunnilingus, douching)
2. Abscess perforation into vessel
3. ARDS
4. Asthmatic episode
5. Decompression sickness (eg, caisson disease)
6. Dental procedure (root canal treatment, drilling)
7. Emphysematous gastritis; corrosive gastritis
8. Gastrointestinal perforation into vessel (eg, enema, peptic ulcer)
9. Hydrogen peroxide enema
10. Injection of gas (eg, cerebral pneumography, arthrography, Rubin's test, artificial pneumothorax or pneumoperitoneum, suicidal or homicidal attempt)
11. Irrigation (lavage) or drainage of abscess, empyema, or paranasal sinus
12. Necrotizing enterocolitis; mesenteric infarction; toxic megacolon

(continued)

13. Neoplasm, malignant, with invasion of vessel (eg, bronchovascular fistula, esophageal-aortic fistula)
14. Sepsis, gas-producing organism (esp. in a diabetic)
15. Thoracentesis, pericardiocentesis, peritoneocentesis (incl. hemodialysis)
16. Whooping cough

References:
1. Cholankeril JV, Joshi RR, Cenizal JS, et al: Massive air embolism from the pulmonary artery. Radiology 1982;142: 33-34
2. Kizer KW, Goodman PC: Radiographic manifestations of venous air embolism. Radiology 1982;144:35-39
3. Kogutt MS: Systemic air embolism secondary to respiratory therapy in the neonate: Six cases including one survivor. AJR 1978;131:425-429
4. Shook DR, Cram KB, Williams HJ: Pulmonary venous air embolism in hyaline membrane disease. AJR 1975;125: 538-542

Gamut C-39

PNEUMOPERICARDIUM

COMMON
1. Iatrogenic (eg, postoperative, intubation, pericardio-centesis, resuscitation, respiratory therapy)

UNCOMMON
1. ARDS
2. Congenital absence of the pericardium with pneumothorax
3. Hyaline membrane disease
4. Idiopathic
5. [Intracardiac gas (See C-38)]
6. Perforation from adjacent abscess (esp. amebic), neoplasm, or radiation necrosis; cutaneous fistula
7. Pericarditis due to gas-forming organism

8. Pneumomediastinum or interstitial pulmonary leakage with extension into pericardium
9. Trauma, external (eg, stab wound, tracheal injury)

Reference:
1. Higgins CB, Broderick TW, Edwards DK, et al: The hemo-dynamic significance of massive pneumopericardium in preterm infants with respiratory distress syndrome. Radiology 1979;133: 363-368

Gamut C-40

CONSTRICTIVE PERICARDITIS

COMMON
1. Idiopathic
2. Tuberculosis

UNCOMMON
1. Asbestosis (pleuropericardial); talcosis
2. Histoplasmosis
3. Neoplasm (eg, primary, metastatic, or locally in-vasive—esp. mesothelioma, malignant thymoma, lymphoma$_g$) (See C-35)
4. Parasitic (eg, amebic abscess from liver or lung rup-turing into pericardial sac)
5. Postpericardiotomy S.
6. Pyogenic infection (esp. staphylococcal, pneumococcal)
7. Radiation therapy
8. Rheumatic
9. Traumatic pericarditis; hemopericardium
10. Uremia
11. Viral pericarditis (esp. Coxsackie B)

(continued)

References:
1. Deutsch V, Miller H, Yahini JH, et al: Angiocardiography in constrictive pericarditis. Chest 1974;65:379-387
2. Elliott LP: Cardiac Imaging in Infants, Children, and Adults. Philadelphia: Lippincott, 1991, pp 373-378
3. Wilson JD, et al: Harrison's Principles of Internal Medicine. (ed 12) New York: McGraw-Hill, 1991

Gamut C-41

PERICARDIAL EFFUSION

COMMON
1. Cardiac failure
2. Collagen disease$_g$ (esp. lupus erythematosus, rheumatoid disease, scleroderma)
3. Neoplasm of pericardium or heart (primary or secondary) (See C-35)
4. Pericarditis (viral, Coxsackie, bacterial, amebic, toxoplasmic, tuberculous, histoplasmic, rheumatic)
5. Postmyocardial infarction S. (Dressler S.)
6. Postpericardiotomy S. (incl. coronary artery bypass)
7. Trauma, external or iatrogenic (hemopericardium)
8. Uremia; nephrotic S.

UNCOMMON
1. Amyloidosis; Waldenström's macroglobulinemia; Mediterranean fever
2. Anemia$_g$ (eg, thalassemia, erythroblastosis fetalis)
3. Behcet S.
4. Beriberi; hypoalbuminemia
5. Bleeding or clotting disorder$_g$ (eg, hemophilia, thrombocytopenia, hypoprothrombinemia)
6. Congenital syndromes (eg, Chester-Erdheim S., Degos S., Kawasaki S., Turner S., Wissler S.)
7. Dissecting aneurysm with leakage
8. Drug reaction

9. Endomyocardial fibrosis (African)
10. Gout
11. Idiopathic
12. Myxedema
13. Pancreatitis
14. Polyserositis
15. Radiation therapy (eg, for lymphoma$_g$, breast or lung cancer)
16. Reiter S.
17. Sarcoidosis
18. Stevens-Johnson S.
19. Superior vena cava obstruction
20. Wegener's granulomatosis
21. Whipple's disease

References:

1. Agner RC, Gallis HA: Pericarditis: Differential diagnostic considerations. Arch Intern Med 1979;139:407-412
2. Taybi H, Lachman RS: Radiology of Syndromes, Metabolic Disorders, and Skeletal Dysplasias. (ed 3) Chicago: Year Book Medical Publ, 1990, pp 831-832
3. Teplick JG, Haskin ME: Roentgenologic Diagnosis. (ed 3) Philadelphia: W.B. Saunders, 1976
4. Wilson JD, et al: Harrison's Principles of Internal Medicine. (ed 12) New York: McGraw-Hill, 1991

Gamut C-42

COMMON CARDIAC CONDITIONS DIAGNOSED BY ECHOCARDIOGRAPHY

1. Aortic stenosis or insufficiency
2. Bacterial endocarditis
3. Cardiac tumor (esp. myxoma of LA)
4. IHSS
5. Mitral stenosis or insufficiency
6. Mitral valve prolapse (MVP)
7. Myocardiopathy

(continued)

8. Pericardial effusion
9. Shunts (with evaluation of flow and direction by pulsed Doppler)

References:

1. Duncan W: Color Doppler in Clinical Cardiology. Philadelphia: W.B. Saunders, 1988
2. Feigenbaum H: Echocardiology. (ed 4) Philadelphia: Lea & Febiger, 1986
3. Goldberg S.: Doppler Echocardiography. (ed 2) Philadelphia: Lea & Febiger, 1988
4. Kisslo J: Doppler Color Flow Imaging. New York: Churchill Livingstone, 1988
5. Seward J, Fajek A, Edwards W, et al: Two Dimensional Echocardiographic Atlas. New York: Springer-Verlag, 1987

Gamut C-43

GENERALIZED PULMONARY ARTERIAL HYPERVASCULARITY
(See Gamuts C-13, C-15)

COMMON
1. High output heart disease (See C-31)
2. Left to right shunt (See C-5)

UNCOMMON
1. Aorta-pulmonary artery fistula (eg, traumatic, postoperative, ruptured aneurysm)
2. Aortic atresia
3. APVR, total
4. Common atrium
5. Cor biloculare
6. Double outlet right ventricle without PS (incl. Taussig-Bing S.)
7. Pulmonary AV malformation
8. Single ventricle without PS

9. Transposition of great vessels with large VSD
10. Tricuspid atresia without PS
11. Truncus arteriosus

References:

1. Elliott LP: Cardiac Imaging In Infants, Children, and Adults. Philadelphia: Lippincott, 1991, p 156
2. Gedgaudas E, Moller JH, Castaneda-Zuniga WR, Amplatz K: Cardiovascular Radiology. Philadelphia: W.B. Saunders, 1985
3. Meszaros WT: Cardiac Roentgenology. Springfield, IL: CC Thomas, 1969, p 324
4. Simon M: The pulmonary vasculature in congenital heart disease. Radiol Clin North Am 1968;6:303-318
5. Swischuk LE: Plain Film Interpretation in Congenital Heart Disease. (ed 2) Baltimore: Williams & Wilkins, 1979
6. Teplick JG, Haskin ME: Roentgenologic Diagnosis. (ed 3) Philadelphia: W.B. Saunders, 1976

Gamut C-44

INCREASED PULMONARY ARTERIAL CIRCULATION TO ONE LUNG

COMMON

1. Air trapping in contralateral lung (eg, Swyer-James S., bullous emphysema)
2. Arteriovenous malformation (congenital or acquired)
3. Obstruction of contralateral pulmonary artery (eg, thromboembolism, neoplasm, histoplasmic lymph-adenopathy)

UNCOMMON

1. Contralateral scimitar S.; hypogenetic lung; pulmonary artery atresia, stenosis, or coarctation
2. Left to right shunt with increased flow to one lung (eg, PDA, AV communis)
3. Postoperative cyanotic congenital heart disease (eg, Waterson, Blalock, or Potts procedure)
4. Unilateral origin of a pulmonary artery from the aorta; truncus arteriosus with single pulmonary artery

(continued)

Reference:
1. Chen JTT, Capp MP, Goodrich JK, et al: Roentgen appearance of pulmonary vascularity in the diagnosis of heart disease. AJR 1971;112:559-570

Gamut C-45

PROMINENCE OF THE MAIN PULMONARY ARTERY SEGMENT

COMMON
1. "Aneurysm" of pulmonary artery (See C-47)
2. Congestive heart failure (See C-4, C-51)
3. Cor pulmonale, pulmonary hypertension, primary or secondary (See C-46)
4. [Enlarged left atrial appendage]
5. High output heart disease (See C-31)
6. Idiopathic
7. Left to right shunt (eg, ASD, VSD, PDA) (See C-5)
8. [Mediastinal or left hilar mass (incl. metastasis)]
9. Mitral stenosis or insufficiency, acquired or congenital
10. Normal (esp. young woman)
11. Pregnancy
12. Pulmonary thromboembolism
13. Pulmonary valvular stenosis (poststenotic dilatation)
14. [Technical or positional factor (eg, lordotic view, patient rotation, cardiac rotation in left lower lobe collapse, dextroscoliosis, pectus excavatum)]

UNCOMMON
1. Absent pulmonary valve
2. Aortopulmonary fistula, postoperative, traumatic or congenital (eg, laceration, ruptured aneurysm, Potts procedure)
3. APVR, partial or total
4. Coarctation of pulmonary artery or its branches

5. Congenital absence of the pericardium
6. Cor triatriatum
7. Double outlet right ventricle
8. Eisenmenger complex
9. Hypoplastic left heart S.$_g$ (incl. interrupted aortic arch)
10. Left to right shunt, other (eg, aorticopulmonary window, atrioventricular canal defect, coronary artery fistula to right heart or PA)
11. Marfan S.
12. Neoplasm of heart (esp. left atrial myxoma) (See C-35)
13. Parachute mitral valve complex
14. Pulmonary insufficiency
15. Tricuspid atresia without pulmonary stenosis
16. Trilogy of Fallot
17. Truncus arteriosus, type 1

References:

1. Burgener FA, Kormano M: Differential Diagnosis in Conventional Radiology. (ed 2) New York: Thieme Medical Publ, 1991, pp 341-345
2. Eisenberg RL: Clinical Imaging: An Atlas of Differential Diagnosis. Rockville, MD: Aspen Publ, 1988, pp 202-205
3. Gedgaudas E, Moller JH, Castaneda-Zuniga WR, Amplatz K: Cardiovascular Radiology. Philadelphia: W.B. Saunders, 1985
4. Meszaros WT: Cardiac Roentgenology. Springfield, IL: CC Thomas, 1969

Gamut C-46

PULMONARY ARTERIAL HYPERTENSION (COR PULMONALE)

CHRONIC HYPOXIA

1. Chest deformity (eg, kyphoscoliosis, thoracoplasty)
2. Chronic upper airway obstruction (eg, enlarged tonsils or adenoids; Crouzon S.)

(continued)

3. High altitude dwelling
4. Neuromuscular disorder$_g$
5. Obesity (Pickwickian S.)
6. Pleural fibrothorax

DIFFUSE LUNG DISEASE
1. Alveolar cell carcinoma
2. Alveolar microlithiasis
3. Bronchiectasis
4. Chronic bronchitis; asthma
5. Collagen disease (eg, scleroderma, rheumatoid lung, lupus erythematosus, dermatomyositis)
6. Congenital syndromes (eg, cutis laxa, Ehlers-Danlos S., Marfan S., Melnick-Needles S.)
7. Cystic fibrosis
8. Emphysema (incl. antitrypsinase deficiency)
9. Fat embolism
10. Histiocytosis X$_g$
11. Interstitial fibrosis
12. Metastases, lymphangitic, embolic (eg, trophoblastic)
13. Pneumoconiosis
14. Sarcoidosis
15. Tuberculosis or fungus disease$_g$

DIFFUSE PULMONARY VASCULAR OR HEART DISEASE
1. Arteritis (eg, polyarteritis nodosa, lupus erythematosus, Takayasu S., Wegener's granulomatosis)
2. Hypoplastic left heart S.$_g$
3. [Idiopathic (usually young women)]
4. Left to right shunt, chronic (esp. ASD, VSD, PDA—Eisenmenger physiology) (See C-5)
5. Left ventricular failure, chronic
6. Mitral stenosis or insufficiency (long-standing)
7. Primary pulmonary hypertension, idiopathic; pulmonary arteriolar sclerosis
8. Pulmonary artery stenoses or coarctations, multiple (incl. Williams S., arteriohepatic dysplasia)

9. Pulmonary thromboembolism (eg, multiple pulmonary emboli, intravenous drug abuse, sickle cell disease, polycythemia vera, tumor emboli)
10. Pulmonary venous hypertension (See C-51)
11. Schistosomiasis
12. Ventriculoatrial shunt for hydrocephalus

References:

1. Fowler NO: The Pericardium in Health and Disease. Mount Kisco, NY: Futura Publishing, 1985
2. Fraser RG, Paré JAP, Paré PD, Fraser RS, Genereux GP: Diagnosis of Diseases of the Chest. (ed 3) Philadelphia: W.B. Saunders, 1988
3. Harvey RM: Pulmonary (arterial) hypertension. In: Clinical Challenges in Cardiopulmonary Medicine, Vol 1. Park Ridge, IL: American College of Chest Physicians
4. Matthay RA, Schwarz MI, Ellis JH Jr, et al: Pulmonary artery hypertension in chronic obstructive pulmonary disease: Determination by chest radiography. Invest Radiol 1981;16:95-100
5. Meszaros WT: Cardiac Roentgenology. Springfield, IL: CC Thomas, 1969, p 78
6. Taybi H, Lachman RS: Radiology of Syndromes, Metabolic Disorders, and Skeletal Dysplasias. (ed 3) Chicago: Year Book Medical Publ, 1990
7. Teplick JG, Haskin ME: Roentgenologic Diagnosis. (ed 3) Philadelphia: W.B. Saunders, 1976

Gamut C-47

PULMONARY ARTERY "ANEURYSM"

COMMON

1. False aneurysm (external trauma, postoperative)
2. Left to right shunt, large (See C-5)
3. Pulmonary arterial hypertension (eg, emphysema, schistosomiasis) (See C-46)
4. Pulmonary valvular stenosis (poststenotic dilatation)

UNCOMMON

1. Arteritis (eg, polyarteritis nodosa, Takayasu S., syphilis)
2. Atherosclerosis

(continued)

3. AV malformation
4. Behcet S.
5. Hughes-Stovin S. (venous thrombosis plus pulmonary artery aneurysms)
6. Idiopathic
7. Medial degeneration or necrosis (eg, Marfan S., Ehlers-Danlos S., mucopolysaccharidoses$_g$, dissection)
8. Mycotic aneurysm (esp. drug addiction)

References:
1. Reid JM, Stevenson JG: Aneurysm of the pulmonary artery. Dis Chest 1959;36:104-107
2. Viamonte M Jr, LePage JR: Pitfalls in the radiographic evaluation of mediastinal abnormalities. Radiol Clin North Am 1968;6:451-465

Gamut C-48

LOCALIZED ENLARGEMENT OF A PULMONARY VESSEL

COMMON
*1. AV malformation, congenital or acquired (eg, traumatic)
2. Obstructed pulmonary vein or artery (eg, thrombus, neoplasm, granulomatous lesion)
*3. Varix, congenital or acquired (eg, mitral stenosis)

UNCOMMON
*1. Aneurysm of pulmonary artery (eg, polyarteritis nodosa, Takayasu S.; mycotic aneurysm in drug addiction)
2. Anomalous insertion site of pulmonary vein into left atrium
3. Anomalous pulmonary vein (eg, scimitar S.); PAPVR
4. Atresia or stenosis of pulmonary vein (veno-occlusive disease)

*5. Bronchial artery dilatation (eg, tetralogy of Fallot)
6. Cirsoid aneurysm
*7. Coarctation or stenosis of pulmonary artery or its branches (poststenotic dilatation)
*8. Mycotic aneurysm of pulmonary artery
9. Sequestration of lung; anomalous pulmonary artery arising from aorta
10. Systemic artery–pulmonary artery shunt (See C-52)
*11. Telangiectasia (eg, portal hypertension, Osler-Weber-Rendu S.)

*Sometimes multiple.

References:

1. Ben-Menachem Y, Kuroda K, Kyger ER III, et al: The various forms of pulmonary varices: Report of three new cases and review of the literature. AJR 1975;125:881-889
2. Lundell C, Finck E: Arteriovenous fistulas originating from Rasmussen aneurysms. AJR 1983;140:687-688
3. Rees S: Arterial connections of the lung: The inaugural Keith Jefferson Lecture. Clin Radiol 1981;32:1-15
4. Taybi H, Lachman RS: Radiology of Syndromes, Metabolic Disorders, and Skeletal Dysplasias. (ed 3) Chicago: Year Book Medical Publ, 1990

Gamut C-49

PULMONARY VALVE OR MAIN PULMONARY ARTERY OBSTRUCTION (OFTEN LEADING TO PULMONARY HYPOVASCULARITY)

COMMON
*1. Lymphadenopathy with compression (eg, sarcoidosis, tuberculosis, histoplasmosis)
*2. Metastatic or locally invasive neoplasm with compression or luminal obstruction (esp. bronchogenic carcinoma, hypernephroma, melanoma, thymoma, lymphoma$_g$)

(continued)

3. Pulmonary valve stenosis or atresia, congenital
*4. Thromboembolism in pulmonary artery

UNCOMMON
*1. Coarctation of pulmonary artery
*2. Compression by aortic aneurysm$_g$
3. Constrictive pericarditis
4. Endomyocardial fibroelastosis
5. Hypertrophy of the left ventricle (Bernheim S.)
6. IHSS; African cardiomyopathy
7. Mediastinal fibrosis
*8. Neoplasm of heart or pulmonary artery (esp. carcinoid, sarcoma, metastatic) (See C-35)
9. Pulmonary stenosis, acquired (eg, rheumatic fever; carcinoid S.)
10. Septal and infundibular hypertrophy from VSD (Gasul S.)
*11. Takayasu S. involving pulmonary artery
12. Tetralogy of Fallot$_g$

*Often unilateral.

References:
1. Fowler NO: The Pericardium in Health and Disease. Mount Kisco, NY: Futura Publishing, 1985
2. Jeffery RF, Moller JH, Amplatz K: The dysplastic pulmonary valve: A new roentgenographic entity; with a discussion of the anatomy and radiology of other types of valvular pulmonary stenosis. AJR 1972;114:322-339
3. Singh D, Tan L: Primary arteritis of the pulmonary vessels and the aorta. Singapore Med J 1975;16:57-61

Gamut C-50

GENERALIZED PULMONARY ARTERIAL HYPOVASCULARITY
(See Gamut C-16)

COMMON

1. Congenital heart disease with right to left shunt (eg, tetralogy or trilogy of Fallot$_g$)
2. Emphysema, diffuse or bullous
3. Pulmonary hypertension, primary or secondary (eg, schistosomiasis)
4. Right ventricular failure, esp. with marked tricuspid insufficiency

UNCOMMON

1. Compression of pulmonary artery trunk (eg, neoplasm, histoplasmic lymphadenopathy)
2. Ebstein's anomaly; Uhl's anomaly
3. Hypoventilation S.
4. Hypovolemia
5. Mechanical obstruction at, or proximal to, tricuspid valve (eg, right atrial myxoma; hypernephroma extending up IVC into RA; tricuspid stenosis)
6. Mitral stenosis (postcapillary hypertension)
7. Myocardiopathy (See C-32)
8. Pericardial tamponade
9. Pulmonary artery stenosis or coarctation
10. Pulmonary valvular stenosis, congenital or acquired (eg, carcinoid)
11. Thromboembolism to many small pulmonary arteries (incl. trophoblastic embolic metastases)
12. Vasculitis (eg, polyarteritis nodosa)

References:
1. Felson B: Chest Roentgenology. Philadelphia: W.B. Saunders, 1973
2. Fraser RG, Paré JAP, Paré PD, Fraser RS, Genereux GP: Diagnosis of Diseases of the Chest. (ed 3) Philadelphia: W.B. Saunders, 1988

(continued)

3. Ravin CE, Cooper C: Review of Radiology. Philadelphia: W.B. Saunders, 1990, p 24
4. Simon M: The pulmonary vasculature in congenital heart disease. Radiol Clin North Am 1968;6:303-318
5. Swischuk LE: Plain Film Interpretation in Congenital Heart Disease. (ed 2) Baltimore: Williams & Wilkins, 1979

Gamut C-51

PULMONARY VENOUS OBSTRUCTION OR HYPERTENSION (INCREASED VENOUS VASCULARITY OR VASCULAR REDISTRIBUTION) (See Gamut C-4)

COMMON
1. Left ventricular failure, any cause (eg, hypertension, myocardial ischemia, high output heart disease) (See C-29, C-30, C-31)
2. Mitral stenosis or insufficiency

UNCOMMON
1. Airway obstruction (eg, laryngeal)
2. Aortic stenosis or insufficiency
3. [Basal emphysema or thromboembolism (redistribution)]
4. Coarctation S. (coarctation of aorta with VSD and/or PDA)
5. Hypoplastic left heart S.$_g$; aortic atresia
6. Myocardiopathy (See C-32)
7. Neoplasm (esp. left atrial myxoma) (See C-35)
8. Obstruction of pulmonary veins
   a. Congenital
      1. APVR, total, (below the diaphragm; or above the diaphragm with stenosis of an anomalous venous trunk)

    2. Atresia or stenosis of the common or individual pulmonary veins

    3. Cor triatriatum

    4. Primary pulmonary veno-occlusive disease

  b. Acquired

    1. Constrictive pericarditis (See C-40)

    2. Mediastinal tumor

    3. Mediastinitis or mediastinal fibrosis (eg, histoplasmosis)

    4. Thrombosis of pulmonary veins

9. Parachute mitral valve complex

10. Peripheral AV malformations

11. Thrombus in left atrium (esp. ball-valve)

References:

1. Chen JTT: Essentials of Cardiac Roentgenology. Boston: Little, Brown, 1987
2. Elliott LP: Cardiac Imaging in Infants, Children, and Adults. Philadelphia: Lippincott, 1991, pp 505-509
3. Lester RG: Radiological concepts in the evaluation of heart disease. Mod Concepts Cardiovasc Dis 1968;37:113-118
4. McLoughlin MJ: Cor triatriatum sinister. Clin Radiol 1970; 21:287-296
5. Meszaros WT: Cardiac Roentgenology. Springfield, IL: CC Thomas, 1969, p 97
6. Robinson AE, Capp MP, Chen JT, et al: Left-sided obstructive diseases of the heart and great vessels. Semin Roentgenol 1968;3:410-419
7. Shackleford GD, Sacks EJ, Mullins JD, et al: Pulmonary veno-occlusive disease: Case report and review of the literature. AJR 1977;128:643-648

Gamut C-52

SYSTEMIC TO PULMONARY VASCULAR SHUNT ON ANGIOGRAPHY
(See Gamut C-19)

COMMON
1. Bronchiectasis
2. Congenital cyanotic heart disease (eg, tetralogy of Fallot$_g$, tricuspid atresia, single ventricle, double outlet right ventricle, complete or corrected transposition of great vessels)
3. Neoplasm of lung (esp. bronchogenic carcinoma)
4. Occlusion of pulmonary artery (eg, thromboembolism, surgical ligation, mediastinal fibrosis, other external compression) (See C-49)
5. Postoperative (eg, Blalock or Potts procedure for tetralogy, Mustard operation for transposition)
6. Sequestration of lung

UNCOMMON
1. Absence or atresia of pulmonary artery
2. Adenomatoid malformation of the lung
3. Anomalous origin of pulmonary artery (eg, right PA from ascending aorta)
4. AV malformation, congenital or acquired (eg, pulmonary, thoracic wall)
5. Cirrhosis of liver
6. Emphysema; chronic bronchitis
7. Infection of chest wall (eg, chronic granuloma of infants, actinomycosis)
8. Neoplasm of thoracic wall (eg, Hodgkin's disease)
9. Occlusion of pulmonary vein
10. Venolobar S.

References:
1. Ekstrom D, Weiner M, Baier B: Pulmonary arteriovenous fistula as a complication of trauma. AJR 1978;130:1178-1180
2. Rees S: Arterial connections of the lung: The inaugural Keith Jefferson Lecture. Clin Radiol 1981;32:1-15

3. Tadavarthy SM, Klugman J, Castaneda-Zuniga WR, et al: Systemic-to-pulmonary collaterals in pathological states. Radiology 1982;144:55-59

Gamut C-53

SMALL ASCENDING AORTA OR AORTIC ARCH

COMMON
1. ASD
2. Coarctation of aorta (long segment infantile type); interrupted aortic arch
3. Decreased cardiac output (eg, endocardial fibroelastosis or other myocardiopathy; small heart; constrictive pericarditis) (See C-32, C-34, C-40)
4. Mitral stenosis or insufficiency
5. [Technical (eg, rotated patient, dextroscoliosis, pectus excavatum)]
6. VSD, large

UNCOMMON
1. APVR, total
2. Atrioventricular canal defect
3. Hypoplastic left heart S.$_g$
4. Supravalvular aortic stenosis (incl. Williams S.)
5. Transposition of great vessels (arch may appear small due to rotation)
6. Tricuspid atresia with transposition

Reference:
1. Meszaros WT: Cardiac Roentgenology. Springfield, IL: CC Thomas, 1969, pp 148-149

Gamut C-54

PROMINENT ASCENDING AORTA OR AORTIC ARCH

COMMON
1. Aneurysm of aorta$_g$
2. Aortic arch anomaly (eg, right aortic arch, double aortic arch)
3. Aortic insufficiency
4. Aortic stenosis (congenital, rheumatic, atherosclerotic)
5. Aortitis (eg, syphilitic, giant cell, rheumatoid, Takayasu's)
6. Atherosclerosis (tortuosity, elongation, unfolding, and/or dilatation of aorta)
7. Coarctation of aorta; pseudocoarctation
8. Hypertensive heart disease
9. Medial degeneration of aorta (eg, Marfan S., Ehlers-Danlos S., other connective tissue disorders) (See C-55A)
10. [Mediastinal mass simulating large aorta (eg, thymoma, lymphoma$_g$, invasive or metastatic carcinoma)]
11. PDA
12. Tetralogy of Fallot$_g$ (incl. pseudotruncus)

UNCOMMON
1. Aneurysm of sinus of Valsalva or coronary artery (See C-56)
2. Aorta–left ventricle tunnel
3. Aortopulmonary window
4. Corrected transposition with left-sided ascending aorta
5. Pulmonary atresia with intact ventricular septum
6. Tricuspid atresia without transposition
7. Truncus arteriosus
8. VSD with reversal of shunt

References:
1. Gedgaudas E, Moller JH, Castaneda-Zuniga WR, Amplatz K: Cardiovascular Radiology. Philadelphia: W.B. Saunders, 1985
2. Liu, YQ: Radiology of aortoarteritis. Radiol Clin North Am 1985;23:671-688
3. Teplick JG, Haskin ME: Roentgenologic Diagnosis. (ed 3) Philadelphia: W.B. Saunders, 1976

Gamut C-55

ANEURYSM OF AORTA AND OTHER MAJOR ARTERIES

COMMON
1. Atherosclerosis
2. Congenital (esp. cerebral—circle of Willis)
3. Dissecting (See C-55A)
4. Trauma (incl. false aneurysm)

UNCOMMON
1. Angiomyolipoma (renal)
2. Cystic medial necrosis (eg, Marfan S.)
3. "Inflammatory" (degenerative abdominal aortic aneurysm with periarterial fibrosis)
4. Mycotic aneurysm (sepsis, bacterial endocarditis, tuberculosis)
5. Necrotizing vasculitis, arteritis (eg, polyarteritis nodosa; lupus erythematosus; Wegener's granulomatosis; drug abuse—esp. metamphetamine; syphilis; Takayasu S.; acute pancreatitis)
6. Neurofibromatosis
7. Osler-Weber-Rendu S.; AV malformation
8. Poststenotic, distal to
   a. Atheromatous stenosis in any vessel
   b. Coarctation in thoracic aorta
   c. Fibromuscular dysplasia (esp. in renal artery)
   d. Subclavian stenosis in thoracic inlet S.
9. Pseudoxanthoma elasticum

(continued)

Reference:
1. Sutton D, Young JWR (eds): A Short Textbook of Clinical Imaging. London: Springer-Verlag, 1990, pp 237-241

Subgamut C-55A

PREDISPOSING CAUSES OF DISSECTING ANEURYSM OF THE ASCENDING AORTA OR ARCH

COMMON
1. Atherosclerosis
2. Coarctation of aorta; bicuspid aortic valve
3. Cystic medial necrosis or degeneration of aorta (esp. Marfan S.)
4. Hypertension
5. Trauma

UNCOMMON
1. Aortic stenosis
2. Cystic medial necrosis, other causes:
   a. Cogan S.
   b. Cutis laxa
   c. Ehlers-Danlos S.
   d. Idiopathic
   e. Mucopolysaccharidoses$_g$
   f. Osteogenesis imperfecta
   g. Polychondritis
   h. Pseudoxanthoma elasticum
   i. Turner S.
3. Infection (eg, bacterial endocarditis—mycotic aneurysm; syphilis)
4. Intramural injection of contrast medium
5. Pregnancy

References:
1. Dow J, Roebuck EJ, Cole F: Dissecting aneurysms of the aorta. Br J Radiol 1970;39:915-927

2. Earnest F IV, Muhm JR, Sheedy PF II: Roentgenographic findings in thoracic aortic dissection. Mayo Clin Proc 1979;54:43-50

3. Meszaros WT: Cardiac Roentgenology. Springfield, IL: CC Thomas 1969, p 160

Gamut C-56

ANEURYSM OF CORONARY ARTERY

COMMON
1. Atherosclerosis
2. Congenital

UNCOMMON
1. Collagen disease$_g$
2. Dissection
3. Iatrogenic (eg, catheter or operative injury)
4. Kawasaki S.
5. Marfan S.
6. Mucopolysaccharidoses$_g$
7. Mycotic (incl. bacterial endocarditis)
8. Necrotizing arteritis
9. Rheumatic heart disease
10. Syphilis
11. Trauma

References:
1. Norwood WI, Miller SW: Case Records of the Massachusetts General Hospital: N Engl J Med 1980;303:571-577
2. Wada J, Endo M, Takao A, et al: Mucocutaneous lymph node syndrome. Chest 1980;77:443-446

Gamut C-57

ARTERIAL STENOSIS AND THROMBOSIS

1. Arteritis (eg, Takayasu's; giant cell; mesenteric)
2. Atherosclerosis with atheromatous plaque
3. Buerger's disease (thromboangiitis obliterans)
4. Congenital lesions (eg, coarctation of thoracic or abdominal aorta, fibromuscular hyperplasia)
5. Extrinsic compression of artery (eg, thoracic inlet S., renal artery stenosis due to fibrous band or neurofibromatosis, popliteal entrapment, celiac compression S.)
6. Neoplastic compression or invasion ("cuffing")

Reference:
1. Sutton D, Young JWR (eds): A Short Textbook of Clinical Imaging. London: Springer-Verlag, 1990, p 244

Gamut C-58

EMBOLUS

COMMON
1. Atheromatous plaque or ulcer with mural thrombus
2. Bacterial endocarditis
3. Iatrogenic (eg, postendarterectomy; arterial or venous catheterization)
4. Septic
5. Venous thrombosis or thrombophlebitis (incl. paradoxical embolus from venous system through patent foramen ovale to systemic circulation)

UNCOMMON
1. Arterial aneurysm with mural thrombus
2. Atrial fibrillation with left atrial thrombus
3. Myocardial infarction with left ventricular thrombus
4. Neoplasm (tumor emboli), incl. left atrial myxoma

ARTERITIS AND OTHER CEREBRAL ARTERIAL DISEASE ON ANGIOGRAPHY (NARROWING, IRREGULARITY, OCCLUSION, OR ANEURYSM)

ARTERITIS

1. Bacterial arteritis, mycotic aneurysm (eg, from abscess, meningitis, osteomyelitis, embolism)
2. Behcet S.
3. Carotid arteritis (infant or child)
4. Collagen disease arteritis (esp. lupus erythematosus)
5. Drug or chemical arteritis (eg, ergot, amphetamine, heroin, arsenic, carbon monoxide)
6. Fungal arteritis (esp. torulosis, actinomycosis, nocardiosis, aspergillosis, phycomycosis)
7. Necrotizing angiitis (eg, polyarteritis nodosa, rheumatic fever, hypersensitivity angiitis, giant cell arteritis, temporal arteritis)
8. Radiation arteritis
9. Rickettsial arteritis
10. Sarcoid arteritis
11. Syphilitic arteritis
12. Takayasu's arteritis
13. Tuberculous arteritis
14. Viral arteritis (eg, herpes zoster)

OTHER CAUSES

1. Arterial spasm (eg, subarachnoid or cerebral hemorrhage; migraine)
2. Arteriosclerosis
3. AV malformation
4. Berry aneurysm
5. Cerebral thrombosis (eg, sickle cell anemia, oral contraceptives)
6. Embolism (eg, subacute bacterial endocarditis, atrial myxoma)
7. Fibromuscular dysplasia (usually extracranial)

(continued)

8. Idiopathic
9. [Increased intracranial pressure]
10. Inflammatory disease of brain (eg, abscess; purulent or tuberculous meningitis)
11. Multiple progressive intracranial artery occlusions with telangiectasia (moyamoya)
12. Neoplasm (eg, glioblastoma, lymphoma$_g$, metastasis)
13. Neurocutaneous syndromes (eg, neurofibromatosis, Sturge-Weber S., tuberous sclerosis)
14. Trauma

References:

1. Ferris EJ, Levine HL: Cerebral arteritis: Classification. Radiology 1973;109:327-341
2. Grainger RG, Allison DJ (eds): Diagnostic Radiology: An Anglo-American Textbook of Imaging. (ed 2) Edinburgh: Churchill Livingstone, 1992, vol 3, pp 1993-1994
3. Hilal SK, Solomon GE, Gold AP, et al: Primary cerebral arterial occlusive disease in children. Radiology 1971;99: 71-94
4. Leeds NE, Rosenblatt R: Arterial wall irregularities in intracranial neoplasms. Radiology 1972;103:121-124

Gamut C-60

EXTRACRANIAL ISCHEMIC LESION SECONDARILY INVOLVING THE BRAIN

COMMON
1. Occlusion or stenosis of brachiocephalic vessels
2. Steal syndromes (eg, subclavian steal) (See C-61)

UNCOMMON
1. Dissecting aneurysm of thoracic aorta
2. Embolization secondary to mitral valve disease or atrial myxoma
3. Takayasu's arteritis

4. Trauma to neck
5. Tumor in neck compromising cervical vessels (eg, thyroid adenoma, neurilemoma)

Reference:
1. Mishkin MM: Extracranial ischemic lesions which secondarily involve the brain. Radiol Clin North Am 1967;5:395-408

Gamut C-61

SUBCLAVIAN STEAL SYNDROME

COMMON
1. Atherosclerosis

UNCOMMON
1. Coarctation of aorta with obliteration of subclavian orifice
2. Extravascular obstruction (eg, fibrous band)
3. Hypoplasia, atresia, or isolation of subclavian artery with anomalous aortic arch
4. Ligation for correction of tetralogy of Fallot or coarctation of aorta
5. Obstruction of subclavian artery secondary to cannulation
6. Vascular ring

References:
1. Becker AE, Becker MJ, Edwards JE, et al: Congenital anatomic potentials for subclavian steal. Chest 1971;60:4-13
2. Massumi RA: The congenital variety of the subclavian steal syndrome. Circulation 1963;28:1149-1152
3. Patel A, Toole JF: Subclavian steal syndrome: Reversal of cephalic blood flow. Medicine 1965;44:289-303

Gamut C-62

AZYGOS VEIN DILATATION*

COMMON

1. Congenital absence or interruption of hepatic segment of inferior vena cava with azygos continuation to SVC (eg, polysplenia S.)
2. Congestive heart failure (eg, right ventricular failure secondary to left ventricular failure or mitral stenosis)
3. Constrictive pericarditis (See C-40)
4. [Enlarged azygos node; mediastinal tumor]
5. Normal (expiration, recumbency)
6. Obstruction of inferior vena cava (See C-64)
7. Obstruction of superior vena cava (See C-63)
8. Overhydration
9. Pericardial effusion (See C-41)
10. Portal hypertension; splenic or portal vein thrombosis
11. Pregnancy
12. Tricuspid insufficiency (See C-22A)

UNCOMMON

1. APVR, total (esp. via the azygos vein)
2. AV malformation (esp. thoracic wall)
3. Idiopathic
4. Mechanical obstruction proximal to or at tricuspid valve (eg, myxoma of RA; hypernephroma extending up IVC into RA; rare tricuspid stenosis)
5. [Right aortic arch with displaced azygos vein]
6. Sequestration of lung (esp. extralobar)
7. Traumatic azygos pseudoaneurysm or AV fistula

* Round or oval density crossing over right main bronchus at the tracheo-bronchial angle and measuring over 10 mm in diameter on erect PA chest radiograph. Azygos vein decreases in size with inspiration, erect position, or Valsalva maneuver.

References:

1. Felson B: Chest Roentgenology. Philadelphia: W.B. Saunders, 1973
2. Fraser RG, Paré JAP, Paré PD, Fraser RS, Genereux GP: Diagnosis of Diseases of the Chest. (ed 3) Philadelphia: W.B. Saunders, 1988

Gamut C-63

SUPERIOR VENA CAVAL DILATATION

COMMON

1. Bronchogenic carcinoma (eg, superior sulcus)
2. Increased central venous pressure (eg, congestive heart failure; cardiac tamponade from pericardial effusion or constrictive pericarditis)
3. Lymphadenopathy (eg, oat cell carcinoma of lung, histoplasmosis, tuberculosis)
4. Lymphoma$_g$
5. Mediastinal fibrosis or granuloma (eg, histoplasmosis, tuberculosis, ergotrate, irradiation, idiopathic)
6. Neoplasm of esophagus, thyroid or mediastinum (eg, goiter, cystic hygroma, thymoma, teratoid tumor)
7. Thrombosis (eg, iatrogenic—broken pacemaker wire, central line catheter, ventriculo-atrial shunt for hydrocephalus, post–tetralogy of Fallot repair; polycythemia vera)

UNCOMMON

1. Aneurysm of aorta or great artery$_g$; AV fistula
2. Axillary vein thrombois with extension
3. Behcet S.
4. Congenital heart disease (eg, tricuspid insufficiency, TAPVR)
5. Idiopathic
6. Mediastinal emphysema, severe; tension pneumothorax
7. Mediastinitis, acute
8. Myxoma of right atrium
9. Osteomyelitis of clavicle
10. Pneumoconiosis (coal-worker's, silicosis) with conglomerate mass
11. Postoperative (eg, after surgery for congenital heart disease)
12. Sarcoidosis
13. Trauma (eg, laceration, transection, mediastinal hematoma)

(continued)

References:
1. Felson B: Chest Roentgenology. Philadelphia: W.B. Saunders, 1973
2. Heitzman ER: The Mediastinum: Radiologic Correlation with Anatomy and Pathology. St. Louis: C.V. Mosby, 1977
3. Mahajan V, Strimlan V, VanOrdstrand HS, et al: Benign superior vena cava syndrome. Chest 1975;68:32-35
4. Mikkelson WJ: Varices of the upper esophagus in superior vena caval obstruction. Radiology 1963;81:945-948
5. Moncada R, Cardella R, Demos TC, et al: Evaluation of superior vena cava syndrome by axial CT and CT phlebography. AJR 1984;143:731-736
6. Scoggin C: Identifying and managing superior vena cava syndrome. J Resp Dis Sept. 1981
7. Shimm DS, Logus MD, Rigsby LC: Evaluating the superior vena cava syndrome. JAMA 1981;245:951-953

Gamut C-64

OBSTRUCTION OF THE INFERIOR VENA CAVA OR ILIAC VEINS

COMMON
1. Direct tumor invasion of IVC (eg, renal cell carcinoma, Wilms' tumor, hepatoma)
2. Extrinsic compression (eg, by lymphadenopathy, retroperitoneal tumor, cyst, hematoma, pelvic lymphocele, aortic aneurysm, liver mass or enlarged liver)
3. Therapeutic interruption of IVC by ligation or filters (eg, to prevent pulmonary emboli, or as therapy for schistosomiasis)
4. Thromboembolism
5. Transient compression (eg, ascites, pregnancy)

UNCOMMON
1. Adhesions
2. [Congenital absence or hypoplasia of IVC]
3. Lymphedema praecox (from compression of left common iliac vein by left common iliac artery)

4. Posttraumatic; post–radiation therapy
5. Retroperitoneal fibrosis
6. Sarcoma of IVC (eg, leiomyosarcoma, angiosarcoma)
7. Web at junction of IVC and RA

Reference:
1. Sutton D, Young JWR: A Short Textbook of Clinical Imaging. London: Springer-Verlag, 1990, p 251

Subgamut C-64A

ANOMALIES OF THE INFERIOR VENA CAVA

1. Absence of IVC	Failure to form a prerenal cava
2. Azygos continuation, unilateral or bilateral	Persistence of left supracardinal vein
3. Bilateral cavae	Failure of dominance of right supracardinal vein
4. Circumaortic venous collar	Failure of regression of superior intersupracardinal anastomosis
5. Left IVC	Regression of right supracardinal vein
6. Retrocaval ureter	Failure of regression of right posterior cardinal vein

Reference:
1. Mayo J, Gray RR, St. Louis EL, et al: Exhibit, American Roentgen Ray Society Meeting, Boston, 1984

ABNORMAL ABDOMINAL VESSELS ON ANGIOGRAPHY

COMMON

1. Aneurysm$_g$
2. Anomalous origin or congenital absence of a vessel (eg, pulmonary sequestration)
3. Arterial occlusion, incl. collateral circulation (eg, via artery of Drummond, arc of Riolan, meandering mesenteric artery)
4. Arteritis, microaneurysms (eg, Behcet S., Takayasu's disease, necrotizing angiitis from drug abuse, mycotic aneurysms, polyarteritis nodosa, other collagen disease$_g$)
5. Atherosclerosis
6. Fibromuscular dysplasia
7. Neoplasm, incl. neovascularity (eg, angiomyolipoma, pheochromocytoma, renal cell carcinoma) or vascular cuffing or displacement (esp. carcinoma)
8. Thromboembolism
9. Trauma (lacerated or transected vessel)
10. Varices (eg, portal venous hypertension or obstruction, inferior vena caval obstruction)

UNCOMMON

1. Anomalous pulmonary vein, draining below the diaphragm (incl. venolobar S.)
2. AV communication
3. Azygos continuation of inferior vena cava
4. Coarctation of abdominal aorta
5. Neurofibromatosis, arterial
6. Phlebitis (esp. pylephlebitis)
7. Portal vein occlusion ("cavernous transformation")
8. Pregnancy (eg, hypertrophied uterine vessels, compression of iliac vein)
9. Pseudoxanthoma elasticum
10. Telangiectasia (eg, Osler-Weber-Rendu S.)

Reference:
1. Moskowitz M, Zimmerman H, Felson B: The meandering mesenteric artery of the colon. AJR 1964;92:1088-1099

Gamut C-66

OBSTRUCTION OF ABDOMINAL LYMPHATIC VESSELS, CISTERNA CHYLI, OR THORACIC DUCT ON LYMPHANGIOGRAPHY (CHYLOUS OR LYMPHATIC ASCITES)

COMMON
1. Lymphoma$_g$
2. Metastasis (esp. lymph node)
3. Neoplasm, benign (esp. lymphangioma)
4. Postoperative
5. Trauma

UNCOMMON
1. Adhesive bands
2. Cirrhosis (hepatic lymphatics visible)
3. [Congenital absence or hypoplasia of lymphatic system]
4. Filariasis
5. Idiopathic
6. Lymphangioleiomyomatosis; tuberous sclerosis
7. Lymphangiomatosis, disseminated (benign metastasizing lymphangiomatosis)
8. Neoplasm compressing or invading lymphatic system (eg, carcinoma of pancreas)
9. Tuberculosis; histoplasmosis

Reference:
1. Griscom NT, Colodny AH, Rosenberg HK, et al: Diagnostic aspects of neonatal ascites: Report of 27 cases. AJR 1977; 128:961-970

Gamut C-67

COMPLICATIONS OF CENTRAL VENOUS (SUBCLAVIAN, JUGULAR) OR PULMONARY ARTERY CATHETERIZATION

COMMON

1. Arterial insertion with perforation (esp. subclavian, carotid artery)
2. Catheter embolism; broken catheter; trapped catheter; occluded catheter
3. Extravascular infusion (eg, mediastinal, intrapleural, subcutaneous)
4. Infection (local or sepsis)
5. Malpositioned or dislodged catheter (eg, in RV, IVC, hepatic vein, jugular vein)
6. Perforation of vessel with hematoma, hemothorax, hydrothorax, hemopericardium, or hemomediastinum
7. Pneumothorax
8. Thrombosis (eg, SVC); thrombophlebitis; pulmonary embolism

UNCOMMON

1. Air embolism
2. AV fistula
3. Cardiac (eg, myocardial perforation, tamponade, arrhythmias)
4. Nerve injury (phrenic or brachial plexus)
5. Subcutaneous or mediastinal emphysema
6. Thoracic duct laceration

References:

1. Boyd KD, Thomas SJ, Gold J, et al: A prospective study of complications of pulmonary artery catheterization in 500 consecutive patients. Chest 1983;84:245-249
2. Gibson RN, Hennessy OF, Collier N, Hemingway AP: Major complications of central venous catheterization; A report of five cases and a brief review of the literature. Clin Radiol 1985; 36:205-208

3. Henschke CI, Pasternack GS, Herman PG: Maximizing the efficacy of chest radiography in the ICU. Appl Radiol, 1984; 13:139-143

4. Kattan KR: Migration of central venous catheters. AJR 1985; 145:727-728

5. Kattan KR, Gutman E, Pantoja E, et al: Tubes, wires and rods seen in chest roentgenograms. CRC Crit Rev Diagn Imag 1984;21:257-287

6. Katz JD, Cronau LH, Barash PG, et al: Pulmonary artery flow-guided catheters in the perioperative period: Indications and complications. JAMA 1977;237:2832-2834

7. Mitchell SE, Clark RA: Complications of central venous catheterization. AJR 1979;133:467-476

8. Wilde P, Hartnell GG: Cardiac tumors; Pericardial tumors. In: Sutton D, Young JWR (eds): A Short Textbook of Clinical Imaging. London: Springer-Verlag, 1990, p 222

Gamut C-68

VASCULAR CALCIFICATION

COMMON

1. Aneurysm
2. Arteriosclerosis
3. Hemangioma; arteriovenous malformation
*4. Hyperparathyroidism, primary or secondary (renal osteodystrophy)
5. Mönckeberg's sclerosis (medial sclerosis)
6. Phleboliths (eg, normal, varicose veins, hemangioma, Maffucci S.)
7. Premature atherosclerosis
    a. Familial hyperlipemia
    b. Generalized (idiopathic) arterial calcification of infancy
    c. Osteogenesis imperfecta tarda
    d. Progeria
    e. Secondary hyperlipemia
        i. Cushing S.
        ii. Diabetes

(continued)

      iii. Glycogen storage disease
      iv. Hypothyroidism
      v. Lipodystrophy
      vi. Nephrotic S.
      vii. Renal homotransplantation
   f. Werner S.

UNCOMMON

1. Buerger's disease
2. Calcified thrombus (eg, vena cava, portal vein, left atrium, pulmonary artery, peripheral artery, Leriche S.)
3. Cystic fibrosis
4. Gout, hyperuricemia
5. Homocystinuria
*6. Hypervitaminosis D
7. Hypoparathyroidism
*8. Idiopathic hypercalcemia (Williams S.)
*9. Immobilization
*10. Milk-alkali S.
11. Ochronosis (alkaptonuria)
12. Oxalosis
13. Pseudoxanthoma elasticum
14. Radiation therapy
15. Raynaud's disease
*16. Sarcoidosis
17. Takayasu's arteritis
18. Thermal injury (eg, burn, frostbite)
*19. Widespread bone destruction (eg, metastatic disease)

* Hypercalcemia.

References:
1. Taybi H, Lachman RS: Radiology of Syndromes, Metabolic Disorders, and Skeletal Dysplasias. (ed 3) Chicago: Year Book Medical Publ, 1990, p 829
2. Teplick JG, Haskin ME: Roentgenologic Diagnosis. (ed 3) Philadelphia: W.B. Saunders, 1976

ROENTGEN SIGNS OF ALVEOLAR DISEASE (CONSOLIDATION, AIR SPACE PATTERN)

1. Acinar or peribronchiolar nodules
2. Air alveologram and bronchiologram
3. Air bronchogram
4. Butterfly or "bat's wing" distribution
5. Coalescence (early)
6. Fluffy, ill-defined margins
7. Present soon after onset of symptoms; rapid change
8. Segmental or lobar distribution

References:
1. Felson B: A new look at pattern recognition of diffuse pulmonary disease. AJR 1979;133:183-189
2. Felson B: Chest Roentgenology. Philadelphia: W.B. Saunders, 1973

PULMONARY EDEMA

COMMON
*1. Agonal
*2. ARDS (eg, shock lung, respirator lung); oxygen toxicity
*3. Aspiration (eg, Mendelson S.)
*4. Cardiac failure (eg, left heart failure, mitral stenosis, total APVR, hypoplastic left heart S., myocardiopathy) (See C-32)
*5. Drug reaction (eg, nitrofurantoin, aspirin, hydrochlorothiazide, beta-adrenergic drugs, interleukin-2, radiologic contrast media)
*6. Glomerulonephritis, acute; nephrosis

(continued)

*7. Iatrogenic (incl. fluid overload, overtransfusion, drug overdose)
8. Narcotics (esp. heroin, morphine, methadone)
9. Neurogenic, cerebral (stroke, head trauma, epilepsy, neoplasm, increased intracranial pressure)
10. Pulmonary infarction, thromboembolism
*11. Renal failure, uremia
12. Sensitivity pneumonitis, extrinsic allergic alveolitis (eg, farmer's lung, silo-filler's disease, bagassosis)

UNCOMMON
*1. Cardiopulmonary bypass, open heart surgery
2. Collagen disease$_g$
*3. Disseminated intravascular coagulopathy
4. Fat embolism (incl. oily contrast medium, amniotic fluid)
*5. Hepatic disease (eg, acute hepatitis)
6. High altitude
*7. Hydrocarbon aspiration
*8. Hypoproteinemia (eg, malabsorption)
*9. Hypoxia, any cause
*10. Inhalation of noxious gas, smoke, paint fumes, sulfur dioxide, beryllium, silica, dinitrogen tetroxide, carbon monoxide, fluorocarbons, hydrocarbons, paraquat, ammonium, chlorine, hydrogen sulfide, phosgene, cadmium
*11. [Lymphangiectasia]
*12. Near-drowning
13. Neoplasm of heart (esp. left atrial myxoma)
14. Pancreatitis, acute
*15. Parasitic disease (eg, malaria, ascariasis, strongyloidiasis)
16. Pericarditis, (esp. constrictive)
17. Pheochromocytoma (catecholamine release)
*18. Pleural air or fluid aspiration, rapid or excessive; reexpansion of lung following treatment for a large pneumothorax
19. Pregnancy
20. Radiation therapy

*21. Shock (eg, insulin reaction; gram negative sepsis; snakebite; electric shock; anaphylactic reaction to penicillin, blood transfusion, or radiologic contrast medium)

*22. Transient tachypnea of newborn (retained fetal lung fluid)

*23. Trauma, thoracic

*24. Upper airway obstruction (eg, aspirated food, foreign body, hanging, suffocation, epiglottitis, croup)

*25. Venous or lymphatic obstruction (eg, pulmonary veno-occlusive disease, blockage by mediastinal mass)

* May occur in an infant.

References:

1. Brodey PA, Fisch AE, Huffaker J: Acute pulmonary edema resulting from treatment for premature labor. Radiology 1981; 140:631-633

2. Fraser RG, Paré JAP, Paré PD, Fraser RS, Genereux GP: Diagnosis of Diseases of the Chest. (ed 3) Philadelphia: W.B. Saunders, 1988

3. Heitzman ER: The Lung: Radiologic-Pathologic Correlations. (ed 2) St. Louis: C.V. Mosby, 1984, p 182

4. Reed JC: Chest Radiology Plain Film Patterns and Differential Diagnoses. (ed 3) St. Louis: Mosby-Year Book, 1991

5. Rigsby C, Swett HA, Sostman HD, et al: Roentgenographic features of drug-induced disease. J Resp Dis 1983;11:60-68

Subgamut C-70A

UNILATERAL PULMONARY EDEMA

COMMON

1. Aspiration, unilateral
2. Contralateral disease (eg, emphysema; occlusion, absence, or hypoplasia of a pulmonary artery — Swyer-James S.)
3. Contusion of one lung

(continued)

4. Idiopathic
5. Postural (prolonged lateral decubitus position)
6. Thoracentesis, too rapid (for pneumothorax or pleural effusion)

UNCOMMON
1. Bronchial obstruction with drowned lung
2. Catheter malposition with infusion into lung
3. Congenital heart disease (eg, unilateral ductus shunt)
4. Postoperative systemic-pulmonary artery shunt (eg, Potts, Blalock, or Waterston operation)

References:
1. Amjad H, Bigman O, Tabor H: Unilateral pulmonary edema. JAMA 1974;229:1094-1095
2. Calenoff L, Kruglik GD, Woodruff A: Unilateral pulmonary edema. Radiology 1978;126:19-24
3. Friedman PJ: Idiopathic and autoimmune type III-like reactions: Interstitial fibrosis, vasculitis, and granulomatosis. Semin Roentgenol 1975;10:43-51
4. Ratliff JL, Chavez CM, Jamchuk A, et al: Re-expansion pulmonary edema. Chest 1973;64:654-656

Gamut C-71

PULMONARY HEMORRHAGE

COMMON
1. Contusion, blunt trauma
2. Renal disease with or without immunologic abnormality (incl. Goodpasture S.)

UNCOMMON
1. Anticoagulant therapy; other drug-induced bleeding
2. Aspiration from a bleeding pulmonary lesion
3. Bleeding or clotting disorder$_g$ (eg, hemophilia, leukemia)

4. Cardiac failure
5. Collagen disease$_g$ (esp. lupus erythematosus)
6. Disseminated intravascular coagulation
7. Drug abuse (esp. heroin)
8. Idiopathic
9. Idiopathic pulmonary hemosiderosis
10. Infection (eg, Rocky Mountain spotted fever, aspergillosis, mucormycosis)
11. Leukocytoclastic vasculitis
12. Mitral stenosis
13. Parasitic disease (esp. strongyloidiasis)
14. Thromboembolism (esp. with infarction)
15. Wegener's granulomatosis

References:

1. Albelda SM, Gefter WB, Epstein DM, et al: Diffuse pulmonary hemorrhage: A review and classification. Radiology 1985;154:289-297
2. Felson B: Chest Roentgenology. Philadelphia: W.B. Saunders, 1973
3. Fiegler VW, Siemoneit KD: Pulmonary manifestations in anaphylactoid purpura (Henoch-Schönlein syndrome). Fortschr Röntgenstr 1981;134:269-272
4. Herman PG, Balikian JP, Seltzer SE, et al: The pulmonary-renal syndrome. AJR 1978;130:1141-1148
5. Reed JC: Chest Radiology. Plain Film Patterns and Differential Diagnoses. (ed 3) St. Louis: Mosby-Year Book, 1991
6. Schwartz EE, Teplick JG, Onesti G, et al: Pulmonary hemorrhage in renal disease: Goodpasture's syndrome and other causes. Radiology 1977;122:39-46

Gamut C-72

ROENTGEN PATTERNS OF INTERSTITIAL DISEASE

1. Bronchial disease (eg, mucoid impaction, bronchiectasis)
2. Discrete miliary nodules
3. Honeycomb lung

(continued)

4. Kerley lines
5. Small irregular shadows (reticular, reticulonodular)
6. Vascular abnormality (incl. pulmonary arterial, pulmonary venous, or bronchial arterial)

References:
1. Felson B: A new look at pattern recognition of diffuse pulmonary disease. AJR 1979;133:183-189
2. Felson B: Disseminated interstitial diseases of the lung. Ann Radiol 1966;9:325-345

Gamut C-73

ACUTE DIFFUSE FINE RETICULAR DENSITIES (KERLEY LINES, ACUTE—A, B, AND C) (See Gamut C-74)

COMMON
1. Pneumonia (esp. interstitial—viral, mycoplasma, pneumocystis)
2. Pulmonary edema (esp. congestive heart failure, uremia, fluid overload, drug reaction) (See C-90)
3. Transient tachypnea of the newborn (retained fetal lung fluid)

UNCOMMON
1. Hypoproteinemia (eg, cirrhosis, nephrosis, burn, exudative skin disorder)
2. Pulmonary hemorrhage (See C-71)
3. Pulmonary veno-occlusive disease, acute
4. Sensitivity pneumonitis (eg, farmer's lung)

References:
1. Felson B: A new look at pattern recognition of diffuse pulmonary disease. AJR 1979;133:183-189

2. Felson B: Chest Roentgenology. Philadelphia: W.B. Saunders, 1973
3. Trapnell DH: The differential diagnosis of linear shadows in chest radiographs. Radiol Clin North Am 1973;11:77-92

Gamut C-74

KERLEY LINES, CHRONIC— A, B, AND C (See Gamut C-73)

COMMON
1. Bronchogenic carcinoma (lymphatic obstruction)
2. Idiopathic
3. Lymphangitic metastases
4. Normal
5. Pneumoconiosis
6. Rheumatic mitral stenosis

UNCOMMON
1. Alveolar proteinosis (late)
2. Bronchiolo-alveolar carcinoma
3. Collagen vascular disease (eg, rheumatoid lung, scleroderma)
4. Congenital heart disease (eg, total APVR)
5. Desquamative interstitial pneumonitis (DIP); lymphocytic interstitial pneumonitis (LIP)
6. Interstitial fibrosis
7. Left atrial neoplasm (esp. myxoma)
8. Lipoid pneumonia$_g$
9. Lymphangiectasia, diffuse
10. Lymphangioleiomyomatosis
11. Lymphoma$_g$ (esp. alveolar); leukemia
12. Mediastinal mass with lymphatic obstruction; sclerosing mediastinitis
13. Pulmonary hemorrhage, late (See C-71)

(continued)

14. Pulmonary veno-occlusive disease
15. Radiation fibrosis
16. Sarcoidosis
17. Thoracic duct ligation, obstruction, or injury

References:
1. Felson B: A new look at pattern recognition of diffuse pulmonary disease. AJR 1979;133:183-189
2. Felson B: Chest Roentgenology. Philadelphia: W.B. Saunders, 1973
3. Heitzman ER: The Lung: Radiologic - Pathologic Correlations. (ed 2) St Louis: CV Mosby, 1984
4. Reed JC: Chest Radiology. Plain Film Patterns and Differential Diagnoses. (ed 3) St. Louis Mosby-Year Book, 1991
5. Trapnell DH: The differential diagnosis of linear shadows in chest radiographs. Radiol Clin North Am 1973;11:77-92

Gamut C-75

LONG LINEAR OR CURVILINEAR SHADOW IN THE LUNG, SOLITARY OR MULTIPLE

COMMON
1. Azygos lobe (rarely hemiazygos lobe on left)
2. Bronchial wall thickening, enlarged bronchus (eg, chronic bronchitis, bronchiectasis—"tram lines")
3. Bulla, pneumatocele, or thin-walled cavity (partially visible)
4. Disk atelectasis, transverse or vertical (Fleischner line)
5. Interlobar fissure, normal or thickened
6. Kerley line
7. Pneumothorax (edge of lung)
8. Pulmonary artery or vein (eg, scimitar S., AV malformation, other anomalous vessel)
9. Scar, linear
10. [Skin fold; artifact]

UNCOMMON

1. Bronchial artery (eg, cyanotic congenital heart disease)
2. Mucoid impaction in bronchus
3. [Pleural band or scar]

References:

1. Fleischner F, Hampton AD, Castleman B: Linear shadows in the lung (interlobar pleuritis, atelectasis and healed infarction). AJR 1941;46:610-618
2. Simon G: Further observations on the long line shadow across a lower zone of the lung. Br J Radiol 1970;43:327-332
3. Trapnell DH: The differential diagnosis of linear shadows in chest radiographs. Radiol Clin North Am 1973;11:77-92

Gamut C-76

BLURRING OF THE HEART BORDER ON PA CHEST FILM

COMMON

1. Idiopathic
2. Infiltrate or edema in lingula, right middle lobe, or anterior segment of an upper lobe
3. Mediastinal lesion, anterior (See C-79)
4. Normal or congested blood vessels (esp. right heart border)
5. Pericardial fat pad
6. Pleural fluid
7. Pleuropericardial adhesion; postinfarction myocardial scar
8. Pneumoconiosis (esp. asbestosis)

UNCOMMON

1. Funnel breast, pectus excavatum
2. Hernia, hepatic
3. Pericarditis, constrictive; mediastinal fibrosis
4. Venolobar S. (areolar tissue)

Reference:

1. Felson B: Chest Roentgenology. Philadelphia: W.B. Saunders, 1973

Gamut C-77

UNILATERAL SMALL HILAR SHADOW

COMMON
1. Air trapping, unilateral
2. Hyperaeration, unilateral
3. Lobar collapse with hilum displaced behind the heart
4. Normal variant
5. Postoperative (eg, lobectomy)
6. Rotation (scoliosis, poor positioning)

UNCOMMON
1. Central pulmonary artery obstruction, unilateral (eg, neoplasm, thromboembolism, histoplasmic lymphadenopathy)
2. Congenital absence, hypoplasia, or coarctation of main pulmonary artery
3. Swyer-James S.

References:
1. Felson B: Chest Roentgenology. Philadelphia: W.B. Saunders, 1973
2. White RI Jr, Kaufman SL, Donner MW: Angiographic diagnosis of venous thromboembolism revisited. Ann Radiol 1980; 23:312-315

Gamut C-78

UNILATERAL HILAR ENLARGEMENT

COMMON
1. Bronchial adenoma (carcinoid)
2. Bronchogenic carcinoma
3. Fungus disease (esp. histoplasmosis, coccidiomycosis, actinomycosis, blastomycosis, sporotrichosis)

4. Lymphoma$_g$
5. Metastasis
6. Pulmonic stenosis, valvular (poststenotic dilatation of left pulmonary artery)
7. Tuberculosis, primary

UNCOMMON
1. Aneurysm of pulmonary artery
2. AV malformation
3. Bronchiolo-alveolar carcinoma
4. Coarctation of a central pulmonary artery (poststenotic dilatation)
5. Cystic fibrosis (mucoviscidosis)
6. Embolus lodged in a main pulmonary artery
7. Infectious lymphadenopathy, other (eg, tularemia, pertussis, mycoplasma, psittacosis)
8. [Mediastinal mass superimposed on hilum (eg, thymoma, bronchogenic cyst)]
9. Obstructed, hypoplastic, or absent contralateral pulmonary artery (eg, neoplasm, histoplasmosis, embolus, Swyer-James S., congenital absence of pulmonary artery)
10. [Pneumonia, juxtahilar]
11. Sarcoidosis

References:
1. Felson B: Chest Roentgenology. Philadelphia: W.B. Saunders, 1973
2. Fraser RG, Paré JAP, Paré PD, Fraser RS: Differential Diagnosis of Diseases of the Chest. Philadelphia: W.B. Saunders, 1991, pp 119-125
3. Heitzman ER: The Mediastinum: Radiologic Correlation with Anatomy and Pathology. St. Louis: C.V. Mosby, 1977
4. Palla A, Donnamaria V, Petruzzelli S, et al: Enlargement of the right descending pulmonary artery in pulmonary embolism. AJR 1983;141:513-517

Gamut C-79

ANTERIOR MEDIASTINAL LESION

Anterior to a curved vertical line extending along the posterior border of the heart and anterior margin of the trachea; on CT or MRI, alongside and anterior to the heart and great vessels

COMMON

*1. Aneurysm of ascending aorta or sinus of Valsalva
 2. Bone lesion (esp. sternum)
 3. [Cardiac enlargement]
 4. Fat deposition (eg, normal epicardial fat pad, Cushing S., steroid therapy, hibernoma, lipomatosis)
*5. Hematoma, hemorrhage (eg, traumatic, bleeding disorder)
 6. Hernia (eg, Morgagni, hepatic)
 7. Innominate or brachiocephalic artery dilatation, buckling or aneurysm
 8. Lymphoma$_g$ (esp. nodular sclerosing Hodgkin's); leukemia
 9. Pericardial cyst
 10. Pericardial disease (eg, effusion, neoplasm, defect)
*11. Teratoid lesion (eg, benign or malignant teratoma, dermoid cyst, seminoma, choriocarcinoma, embryonal cell carcinoma)
*12. Thymic lesion (eg, benign or malignant thymoma, thymic cyst, thymolipoma, lymphoma or leukemia arising in thymus, carcinoid tumor)
 13. Thymus, normal ("hyperplasia")
*14. Thyroid mass (intrathoracic goiter, adenoma, carcinoma)

UNCOMMON

 1. Anomalous left superior vena cava
 2. Bronchogenic cyst

*3. Cardiac lesion (eg, tumor, aneurysm)
 4. Cystic hygroma (lymphangioma)
 5. Giant lymph node hyperplasia (Castleman's disease)
 6. Hydatid cyst
 7. Mediastinitis_g, acute; mediastinal abscess
*8. Mediastinitis, chronic sclerosing (esp. histoplasmosis)
 9. Metastasis
*10. Neoplasm, other (eg, spindle cell tumor_g, lipoma, hemangioma, and their sarcomatous counterparts; mesothelioma)
 11. Paraganglioma (chemodectoma, pheochromocytoma); neurofibroma
 12. Parathyroid adenoma, carcinoma
*13. Sarcoidosis
 14. Superior vena caval dilatation (See C-63)

* May show calcification.

References:

1. Daniel RA Jr, Diveley WL, Edwards WH, et al: Mediastinal tumors. Ann Surg 1960;151:783-795
2. Felson B: Chest Roentgenology. Philadelphia: W.B. Saunders, 1973
3. Fraser RG, Paré JAP, Paré PD, Fraser RS, Genereux GP: Diagnosis of Diseases of the Chest. (ed 3) Philadelphia: W.B. Saunders, 1988
4. Heitzman ER: The Mediastinum: Radiologic Correlations with Anatomy and Pathology. St. Louis: C.V. Mosby, 1977
5. Reed JC: Chest Radiology. Plain Film Patterns and Differential Diagnoses. (ed 3) St. Louis: Mosby-Year Book, 1991, pp 97-108
6. Rosenow EC III, Hurley BT: Disorders of the thymus. A review. Arch Intern Med 1984;144:763-770
7. Silverman FN (ed): Caffey's Pediatric X-ray Diagnosis. (ed 8) Chicago: Year Book Medical Publ, 1985

Gamut C-80

MIDDLE MEDIASTINAL LESION

Between anterior and posterior mediastinum on plain film, CT, or MRI

COMMON
*1. Aneurysm of aorta or major artery$_g$ (incl. traumatic, mycotic)
 2. Arygos vein or SVC dilatation
*3. Duplication cyst$_g$ (eg, bronchogenic, tracheal, enteric)
 4. Esophageal lesion (eg, achalasia; diverticulum; spindle cell neoplasm$_g$, esp. leiomyoma)
 5. Hiatal hernia
*6. Lymph node enlargement (eg, metastasis, lymphoma$_g$, tuberculosis, histoplasmosis, sarcoidosis)
 7. Mediastinitis, chronic sclerosing (esp. histoplasmosis)
 8. Pulmonary artery dilatation
 9. Right aortic arch, vascular ring (See C-18)
*10. Thyroid mass (intrathoracic)
 11. Varices, mediastinal or esophageal

UNCOMMON
 1. Chemodectoma (aorticopulmonary paraganglioma)
 2. Cystic hygroma (lymphangioma)
 3. Extramedullary hematopoiesis
 4. Giant lymph node hyperplasia (Castleman's disease)
 5. Mediastinal hematoma or hemorrhage
 6. Mediastinitis$_g$, acute; mediastinal abscess
 7. Neoplasm, mediastinal (eg, spindle cell tumor$_g$, lipoma, hemangioma, mesothelioma)
 8. Neurinoma, vagus or phrenic
 9. Pancreatic pseudocyst
 10. Parathyroid tumor
 11. Sequestration, extralobar (incl. esophageal lung)
 12. Tracheal tumor
 13. Vascular lesion, other (eg, left superior vena cava, aberrant right subclavian artery, angiosarcoma of pulmonary artery)

References:
1. Daniel RA Jr, Diveley WL, Edwards WH, et al: Mediastinal tumors. Ann Surg 1960;151:783-795
2. Felson B: Chest Roentgenology. Philadelphia: W.B. Saunders, 1973
3. Heitzman ER: The Mediastinum: Radiology Correlations with Anatomy and Pathology. St. Louis: C.V. Mosby, 1977
4. Reed JC: Chest Radiology. Plain Film Patterns and Differential Diagnoses. (ed 3) St. Louis. Mosby Year Book, 1991, pp 109-129
5. Reed JC, Sobonya RE: Morphologic analysis of foregut cysts in the thorax. AJR 1974;120:851-860
6. Silverman FN (ed): Caffey's Pediatric X-Ray Diagnosis. (ed 8) Chicago: Year Book Medical Publ, 1985

Gamut C-81

CT OF MEDIASTINAL LESIONS CLASSIFIED ACCORDING TO THEIR DENSITY

FAT DENSITY (-20 to -100 HU)
*1. Dermoid cyst (cystic teratoma)
 2. Hernia (eg, omental, mesenteric)
*3. Lipoma, liposarcoma, hibernoma (incl. thoracoabdominal)
 4. Lipomatosis (Cushing S., steroid therapy, obesity, diabetes)
 5. Normal fat (eg, epicardial fat pad, intrapericardial fat)
 6. Thymolipoma

WATER DENSITY (0-15 HU)
*1. Cyst (eg, bronchogenic, gastroenteric, neurenteric; dermoid; thymic; pericardial; hydatid)
 2. Esophageal dilatation
 3. Lymphocele
 4. Meningocele, meningomyelocele
 5. Pancreatic pseudocyst

(continued)

6. Pleural or pericardial effusion, loculated
*7. Solid neoplasm with cystic degeneration (eg, cystic thymoma, neurogenic tumor)

SOFT TISSUE DENSITY (15-40 HU)

*1. Cardiac neoplasm (See C-35)
 2. Esophageal neoplasm
 3. Extramedullary hematopoiesis
*4. Hematoma
 5. Hernia (hepatic, Morgagni, hiatal, Bochdalek)
*6. Lymphadenopathy (incl. Castleman's disease)
 7. Lymphangioma
 8. Lymphoma$_g$
 9. Mediastinal hemorrhage or hematoma
10. Mediastinitis$_g$, acute; mediastinal abscess; chronic mediastinitis
11. Metastasis
*12. Neurogenic tumor$_g$
13. Parathyroid neoplasm
*14. Sequestration, extralobar
15. Spindle cell tumor$_g$
*16. Teratoid lesion
17. [Thoracic kidney]
18. Thymic hyperplasia
*19. Thymoma
*20. Thyroid goiter or neoplasm

CALCIFICATION*

 1. Aneurysm
 2. Bronchogenic cyst
 3. Dermoid cyst, teratoma
 4. Hemangioma (phleboliths)
 5. Hematoma, old
 6. Lipoma
 7. Lymph nodes
 8. Neurogenic tumor with cystic degeneration
 9. Thymoma, esp. with cystic degeneration
10. Thyroid goiter

VASCULAR OR ENHANCING

*1. Aneurysm, aorta or other (incl. dissection)
2. Azygos dilatation
3. Benign lymphoid hyperplasia (Castleman's disease)
4. Carcinoid
*5. Hemangioma
6. Intrathoracic goiter; thyroid malignancy
7. Paraganglioma
8. Parathyroid adenoma
9. Vessels (varices, collaterals, ectatic vessels, vascular anomalies)

* May show calcification.

References:

1. Brunner DR, Whitley NO: A pericardial cyst with high CT numbers. AJR 1984;142:279-280
2. Chalaoui J, Sylvestre J, Dussault, et al: Thoracic fatty lesions: Some usual and unusual appearances. J Can Assoc Radiol 1981;32:197-201
3. Eisenberg RL: Clinical Imaging: An Atlas of Differential Diagnosis. (ed 2) Rockville, MD: Aspen Publishers, 1992, pp 108-129
4. Mendelson DS, Rose JS, Efremidis SC, et al: Bronchogenic cysts with high CT numbers. AJR 1983;140:463-465
5. Mendez G Jr, Isikoff MB, Isikoff SK, et al: Fatty tumors of the thorax demonstrated by CT. AJR 1979;133:207-212
6. Pugatch RD, Braver JH, Robbins AH, et al: CT diagnosis of pericardial cysts. AJR 1978;131:515-516

Gamut C-82

WIDENING OF THE MEDIASTINUM

COMMON

1. Achalasia; Chagas' disease
2. Hematoma or hemorrhage (eg, sternal or vertebral fractures; venous and arterial tears; aortic transection; postoperative; malposition of vascular catheter with vessel injury)
3. Hiatal hernia, large

(continued)

4. Lymphadenopathy
5. Mediastinitis
6. Neoplasm (eg, primary mediastinal tumor or cyst, lymphoma$_g$, metastatic disease, esp. from lung or esophageal carcinoma)
7. [Technical factors (eg, expiration or poor inspiration, rotation, AP supine or lordotic film)]
8. Vascular abnormality (eg, dilated or tortuous aorta; aneurysm, dissection or coarctation of aorta; congenital left superior vena cava; dilated SVC)

UNCOMMON
1. Allergic edema of mediastinum
2. Chylomediastinum (eg, thoracic duct obstruction or laceration)
3. Extension of extrathoracic infection (eg, pharyngeal or abdominal abscess, pancreatitis, or pancreatic pseudocyst)
4. Extramedullary hematopoiesis
5. Lipomatosis (eg, obesity, steroid therapy, Cushing S., normal variant)
6. Penetrating trauma (eg, knife or gunshot wound)
7. Pleural disease adjacent to mediastinum (eg, metastatic disease, mesothelioma, effusion)

Reference:
1. Reed JC: Chest Radiology. Plain Film Patterns and Differential Diagnoses. (ed 3) St. Louis: Mosby-Year Book, 1991, pp 83-96

Gamut C-83

RIGHT ANTERIOR CARDIOPHRENIC ANGLE LESION

COMMON
1. Epicardial fat pad ("lipoma")
2. [Localized paralysis of right hemidiaphragm ("partial eventration")

3. Morgagni hernia (gut or omentum)
4. Pericardial cyst or diverticulum
5. Pleural effusion, encapsulated; pleural adhesions
6. Right middle lobe disease (eg, neoplasm, pneumonia, atelectasis)

UNCOMMON
1. Cardiac aneurysm or neoplasm
2. Diaphragmatic neoplasm
3. Fat pad necrosis
4. Herniation of liver, traumatic or congenital ("ectopic lobe")
5. Hydatid cyst (cardiac, pericardial, or pulmonary)
6. Lymph node enlargement, juxtapericardial (esp. lymphoma$_g$)
7. Mediastinal mass, anterior (esp. thymic or teratoid lesion, lymphoma$_g$) (See C-79)
8. Mesothelioma, pleural or pericardial
9. Metastasis
10. Pericardial effusion, encapsulated
11. [Right atrial dilatation]

References:

1. Castellino RA, Blank N: Adenopathy of the cardiophrenic angle (diaphragmatic) lymph nodes. AJR 1972;114:509-515
2. Felson B: Chest Roentgenology. Philadelphia: W.B. Saunders, 1973
3. Fraser RG, Paré JAP, Paré, Fraser RS, Genereux GP: Diagnosis of Diseases of the Chest. (ed 3) Philadelphia: W.B. Saunders, 1988

Gamut C-84

RETROCARDIAC LESION IN A CHILD

COMMON
1. Atelectasis of lower lobe
2. Hernia, diaphragmatic (eg, hiatal, Bochdalek, traumatic)

(continued)

3. [Left atrial enlargement]
4. Lymphadenopathy
5. Mediastinal lesion, middle or posterior (See C-80)
6. Pleural effusion
7. Pneumonia or other lower lobe disease
8. Sequestration of lung
9. Spinal disease, paraspinal lesion

UNCOMMON
1. Azygos vein dilatation
2. Pulmonary neoplasm or cyst

Gamut C-85

PLEURAL EFFUSION WITH NORMAL LUNG
(See Gamut C-86)

COMMON
1. Abscess, subphrenic or hepatic (eg, amebic, pyogenic)
2. Asbestos related pleural disease
3. Ascites with permeation of diaphragm (eg, cirrhosis; Meigs S.; peritoneal metastases; extension of retroperitoneal urine collection; peritoneal dialysis)
4. Collagen vascular disease$_g$ (esp. lupus erythematosus, rheumatoid disease)
5. Congestive heart failure (esp. posttreatment)
6. Idiopathic
7. Infection, other (eg, bacterial, viral, infectious mononucleosis, mycoplasma, actinomycosis, nocardiosis)
8. Lymphoma$_g$, mediastinal or retroperitoneal; leukemia
9. Metastasis to pleura (esp. from breast, pancreas, GI tract, ovary, kidney)
10. Normal, physiologic (up to 5 cc); pregnancy

11. Postmyocardial infarction S. (Dressler S.); postpericardiotomy S.
12. Postoperative, following thoracic, abdominal, or retroperitoneal surgery (eg, splenectomy, renal surgery)
13. Thromboembolism of lung
14. Trauma to chest wall, great vessels, thoracic duct (blood, lymph)
15. Tuberculosis

UNCOMMON

1. Bleeding or clotting disorder$_g$
2. Chest wall neoplasm (eg, Ewing's sarcoma, osteo-sarcoma, chondrosarcoma)
3. Constrictive pericarditis
4. Drug reaction (eg, methysergide, nitrofurantoin, busulfan, bromcriptine, procarbazine; also lupus reaction from Dilantin, hydralazine, isoniazid, procainamide, propylthiouracil)
5. Empyema from retropharyngeal or neck abscess, or in postpneumonectomy space
6. Esophageal rupture
7. Familial recurring polyserositis (Mediterranean fever)
8. Hypoproteinemia (incl. hepatic failure)
9. Iatrogenic (eg, ventriculopleural or other shunt, im-properly inserted intravenous catheter, instillation of medication)
10. Lymphothorax (eg, lymphedema, Milroy's disease) (See C-88)
11. Mesothelioma of pleura
12. Multiple myeloma
13. Myxedema
14. Pancreatitis; pancreatic pseudocyst, abscess, or neoplasm
15. Parasitic disease (eg, amebiasis, paragonimiasis, malaria)
16. Pleural fistula (eg, gastric, esophageal, bronchial)
17. Radiation therapy
18. Renal disease (eg, renal failure, nephrosis, acute glomerulonephritis, hydronephrosis, uremic pleuritis)

(continued)

References:
1. Baron RL, Stark DD, McClennan BL: Intrathoracic extension of retroperitoneal urine collection. AJR 1981;137:37-41
2. Eisenberg RL: Clinical Imaging: An Atlas of Differential Diagnosis. (ed 2) Rockville, MD: Aspen Publishers, 1992, pp 144-147
3. Fraser RG, Paré JAP, Paré PD, Fraser RS: Differential Diagnosis of Diseases of the Chest. Philadelphia: W.B. Saunders, 1991, pp 99-106
4. Reed JC: Chest Radiology. Plain Film Patterns and Differential Diagnoses. (ed 3) St. Louis: Mosby-Year Book, 1991, pp 37-49
5. Rosenow EC III: The spectrum of drug-induced pulmonary disease. Ann Intern Med 1972;97:977-991
6. Storey DD, Dines DE, Coles DT: Pleural effusion: A diagnostic dilemma. JAMA 1976;236:2183-2186
7. Teplick JG, Haskin ME: Roentgenologic Diagnosis. (ed 3) Philadelphia: W.B. Saunders, 1976

Gamut C-86

PLEURAL EFFUSION WITH RADIOGRAPHIC EVIDENCE OF OTHER DISEASE IN THE CHEST
(See Gamut C-85)

COMMON
1. Abscess, pulmonary or subphrenic
2. Bronchogenic carcinoma
3. Congestive heart failure
4. Metastasis (esp. from lung, breast, pancreas, or GI tract)
5. Pneumonia (esp. bacterial, usually with empyema—staphylococcal, streptococcal, klebsiella, plague, tularemia)
6. Postoperative (eg, pneumonectomy)
7. Pulmonary embolism and infarction
8. Trauma, esp. laceration of lung, pulmonary or mediastinal hematoma, aortic rupture, or esophageal perforation (blood, lymph, or chyle)
9. Tuberculosis

UNCOMMON

1. Asbestosis
2. Bronchopleural fistula
3. Collagen disease$_g$ (esp. lupus erythematosus, rheumatoid disease)
4. Constrictive pericarditis
5. Drug-induced pulmonary disease, usually diffuse interstitial (eg, nitrofurantoin, hydralazine, procainamide)
6. Eosinophilic pneumonia$_g$
7. Infection, other (eg, fungal, actinomycosis, nocardiosis, mycoplasma, viral)
8. Lymphangioleiomyomatosis; tuberous sclerosis
9. Lymphoma$_g$
10. Malignant neoplasm, other (eg, bronchiolo-alveolar carcinoma, mesothelioma, multiple myeloma, chest wall tumor)
11. Obstruction of superior vena cava or azygos vein
12. Parasitic disease (eg, amebiasis, paragonimiasis, hydatid disease)
13. Radiation therapy
14. Sarcoidosis
15. Uremia (with pulmonary edema)
16. Waldenström's macroglobulinemia
17. Wegener's granulomatosis$_g$

References:

1. Baron RL, Stark DD, McClennan BL: Intrathoracic extension of retroperitoneal urine collection. AJR 1981;137:37-41
2. Eisenberg RL: Clinical Imaging: An Atlas of Differential Diagnosis. (ed 2) Rockville, MD: Aspen Publishers, 1992, pp 148-151
3. Fraser RG, Paré JAP, Paré PD, Fraser RS: Differential Diagnosis of Diseases of the Chest. Philadelphia: W.B. Saunders, 1991, pp 107-118
4. Reed JC: Chest Radiology. Plain Film Patterns and Differential Diagnoses. (ed 3) St. Louis: Mosby-Year Book, 1991, pp 37-49
5. Storey DD, Dines DE, Coles DT: Pleural effusion. A diagnostic dilemma. JAMA 1976;236:2183-2186
6. Teplick JG, Haskin ME: Roentgenologic Diagnosis. (ed 3) Philadelphia: W.B. Saunders, 1976

PLEURAL EFFUSION WITH ENLARGED CARDIAC SILHOUETTE

1. Collagen vascular disease$_g$ (esp. lupus erythematosus, rheumatoid disease)
2. Congestive heart failure
3. Malignant neoplasm with direct or metastatic extension to pleura and heart (eg, mesothelioma, malignant thymoma, carcinoma of lung or esophagus)
4. Myocardiopathy
5. Myocarditis or pericarditis with pleuritis (eg, tuberculosis, rheumatic fever, viral infection)
6. Postpericardiotomy S. (esp. CABG)
7. Pulmonary embolism

Reference:

1. Reed JC: Chest Radiology. Plain Film Patterns and Differential Diagnoses. (ed 3) St. Louis: Mosby-Year Book, 1991, p 41

MASSIVE PLEURAL EFFUSION

COMMON

1. Ascites (leaky diaphragm)
2. Congestive heart failure
3. Empyema; perforated subphrenic or liver abscess
4. Hemothorax (eg, traumatic; bleeding disorder$_g$)
5. Metastatic disease
6. Nephrosis
7. Postoperative
8. Tuberculosis

UNCOMMON

1. Fungus disease
2. Iatrogenic (eg, perforation by venous catheter)

---

3. Idiopathic
4. Lymphoma$_g$
5. Lymphothorax (See C-88)
6. Mesothelioma of pleura, malignant
7. Perforation of esophagus or stomach
8. Polyserositis
9. Pulmonary infarction

References:

1. Liberson M: Diagnostic significance of the mediastinal profile in massive unilateral pleural effusions. Am Rev Resp Dis 1963;88:176-180
2. Swischuk LE: Differential Diagnosis in Pediatric Radiology. Baltimore: Williams & Wilkins, 1984

Gamut C-88

CHYLOTHORAX, LYMPHOTHORAX

COMMON

1. Iatrogenic (esp. surgical or catheter injury to thoracic duct)
2. Idiopathic
3. Neoplasm involving thoracic duct or mediastinum (eg, lymphoma$_g$, carcinoma of esophagus or lung, intrathoracic thyroid)
4. Trauma to thoracic duct

UNCOMMON

1. Aneurysm of thoracic duct with rupture
2. Cirrhosis of liver
3. Congenital anomaly (eg, atresia or fistula of thoracic duct; yellow nail S.; Noonan S.)
4. Filariasis
5. Lymphadenopathy (eg, tuberculous, fungal, other infection)
6. Lymphangioleiomyomatosis
7. Lymphangioma

(continued)

8. Mass, nonneoplastic, compressing the thoracic duct (eg, aortic aneurysm$_g$, spinal disease)
9. Nephrosis
10. Thromboembolism of left subclavian or innominate vein, or superior vena cava

References:
1. Bower GC: Chylothorax: Observations in 20 cases. Chest 1964;46:464-468
2. Freundlich IM: The role of lymphangiography in chylothorax. A report of six nontraumatic cases. AJR 1975;125:617-627
3. Hesseling PG, Hoffman H: Chylothorax: A review of the literature and report of 3 cases. S Afr Med J 1981;60:675-678
4. Hughes RL, Mintzer RA, Hidvagi DF, et al: The management of chylothorax. Chest 1979;76:212-218

Gamut C-89

CLASSIFICATION OF RIB NOTCHING

ARTERIAL

1. High aortic obstruction
   a. Coarctation of aorta
2. Low aortic obstruction
   a. Aortic thrombosis
3. Subclavian obstruction
   a. Blalock-Taussig procedure (unilateral)
   b. Pulseless disease (eg, Takayasu's arteritis); advanced arteriosclerosis
4. Pulmonary oligemia
   a. Absent pulmonary artery (unilateral)
   b. Ebstein's anomaly
   c. Emphysema
   d. Pseudotruncus arteriosus
   e. Pulmonary valvular stenosis or atresia
   f. Tetralogy of Fallot$_g$

VENOUS
1. Obstruction of superior vena cava, innominate or sub-clavian vein

ARTERIOVENOUS
1. A-V fistula of chest wall (intercostal artery-vein)
2. Pulmonary A-V fistula

NEUROGENIC
1. Intercostal neurofibroma or neurilemoma
2. Neurofibromatosis
3. Bulbar poliomyelitis; quadriplegia

OSSEOUS
1. Hyperparathyroidism
2. Osteodysplasty (Melnick-Needles S.)
3. Thalassemia

MISCELLANEOUS
1. Idiopathic; normal variant
2. Indwelling catheter

References:
1. Boone ML, Swenson BE, Felson B: Rib notching: Its many causes. Am J Roentgenol 1964;91:1075-1088
2. Felson B, Weinstein AW, Spitz HB: Principles of Chest Roentgenology: A Programmed Text. Philadelphia: W.B. Saunders, 1965, p 197

Gamut C-90

DISEASES COMMON TO THE TROPICS AND DEVELOPING COUNTRIES THAT MAY INVOLVE THE CARDIOVASCULAR SYSTEM*

HEART

1. Amebiasis (pneumopericardium after abscess rupture)
2. Aneurysms (subvalvular or idiopathic aortic)
3. Aortitis, idiopathic
4. Burkitt's lymphoma
5. Cardiomegaly (idiopathic, puerperal)
6. Chagas' disease
7. Cysticercosis
8. Endomyocardial fibrosis
9. Hemoglobinopathies
10. Hydatid disease
11. Hypertension, systemic or pulmonary (eg, secondary to schistosomiasis)
12. Kwashiorkor, malnutrition
13. Tuberculosis

PERICARDIAL EFFUSION

1. Amebiasis
2. Hemoglobinopathies
3. Hydatid disease
4. Kaposi's sarcoma
5. Malignant disease
6. Rheumatic fever
7. Tuberculosis
8. Viral disease

AORTA, PULMONARY ARTERIES, PERIPHERAL ARTERIES AND VEINS

1. Idiopathic arteritis (Takayasu's disease); aneurysms
2. Peripheral vascular disease; idiopathic gangrene; varicose veins

3. Pulmonary embolus and infarction
4. Pulmonary hypertension (secondary to schistosomiasis)

* When searching for the differential diagnosis of an abnormal cardiovascular finding on a radiograph of a patient or visitor from the tropics, it will be helpful to consult this list, which refers to the major parasitic, infectious, neoplastic, and other diseases that can affect the cardiovascular system.

Reference:

1. Reeder MM, Palmer PES: The Radiology of Tropical Diseases, with Epidemiological, Pathological and Clinical Correlation. Baltimore: Williams & Wilkins, 1981, pp XV- XVIII

Abbreviations

AIDS	acquired immune deficiency S.
AP	anteroposterior
APVR	anomalous pulmonary venous return, total (T) or partial (P)
ARDS	adult respiratory distress syndrome
ASD	atrial septal defect
AV	atrioventricular (communis or canal)
AV(M)	arteriovenous (malformation)
CABG	coronary artery bypass graft
CNS	central nervous system
COPD	chronic obstructive pulmonary disease
eg	for example
esp	especially
g	consult Glossary
HIV	human immunodeficiency virus
IHSS	idiopathic hypertrophic subaortic stenosis
ie	that is
incl	including
IVC	inferior vena cava
L	left
LA	left atrium
LV	left ventricle
occas	occasionally
PA	posteroanterior
PDA	patent ductus arteriosus
PEEP	positive end-expiratory pressure
PS	pulmonary stenosis
pulm	pulmonary
R	right
RA	right atrium
RV	right ventricle
S.	syndrome
SVC	superior vena cava
vasc	vasculature
VATER S.	vertebral (or vascular) anomalies; anal anomalies (or auricular defects); tracheoesophageal fistula; esophageal atresia (or ring); renal anomalies (or radial defects, rib anomalies)
VSD	ventricular septal defect

Glossary

ANEMIA, PRIMARY - erythroblastosis, hemolytic anemia, pyruvate kinase deficiency, sickle cell disease and variants, spherocytosis, thalassemia and variants

ANEURYSM - arteriosclerotic, arteriovenous (incl. fistula, malformation), dissecting, false, mycotic, poststenotic, syphilitic (See ANGIOMA)

ANGIOMA - arteriovenous malformation, cirsoid aneurysm, hemangioma (incl. capillary, cavernous), varices

ARDS - adult respiratory distress syndrome, shock lung, respirator lung, adult hyaline membrane disease, and many other synonyms: a confusing term, widely used and poorly defined, associated with widespread pulmonary involvement

ARTERIOSCLEROTIC HEART DISEASE - coronary heart disease

ARTERIOVENOUS MALFORMATION (AVM) - See ANEURYSM, ANGIOMA

BLEEDING OR CLOTTING DISORDER - anticoagulant effect, coagulopathy (eg, disseminated intravascular type-DIC), hemophilia, purpura (eg, Henoch-Schönlein), thrombocytopenia

COLLAGEN DISEASE - dermatomyositis, lupus erythematosus, polyarteritis nodosa, scleroderma, mixed connective tissue disease (MCTD), CREST S. (calcinosis-Raynaud's- sclerodactyly-telangiectasia)

GLYCOGEN STORAGE DISEASE - von Gierke (Type I), Pompe (Type II), Cori (Type III), McArdle (Type V)

HYPOPLASTIC LEFT HEART SYNDROME - includes aortic stenosis or atresia, cor triatriatum, hypoplastic aorta, hypoplastic left ventricle, interrupted aortic arch, infantile coarctation, severe mitral stenosis or atresia

LYMPHOMA - includes angioimmunoblastic lymphadenopathy, Burkitt's lymphoma, Hodgkin's disease, non-Hodgkin's lymphoma, leukemia (all varieties, including chloroma), pseudo-lymphoma, Sézary S.

MEDIASTINITIS - abscess, cellulitis, edema, fibrosis, granuloma, phlegmon

MUCOPOLYSACCHARIDOSES - also mucolipidoses and other lysosomal storage diseases

NEUROMUSCULAR DISORDERS - amyotonia congenita, amyotrophic lateral sclerosis, cerebral palsy, Duchenne S., meningomyelocele, muscular dystrophy, myasthenia gravis, myotonic dystrophy, parkinsonism, poliomyelitis, visceral myopathy, Werdnig-Hoffmann disease

SPINDLE CELL NEOPLASM - fibroma, leiomyoma, neurofibroma, rhabdomyoma, and their malignant counterparts

TETRALOGY OF FALLOT - include also pentalogy (tetralogy plus ASD), pseudotruncus arteriosus, pulmonary atresia with VSD and systemic pulmonary collateral arteries, trilogy of Fallot (pulmonary stenosis with ASD)

THYROID MASS - adenoma, goiter, intrathoracic goiter (substernal, retrosternal), struma, thyroiditis

VASCULAR RING - aberrant right subclavian artery, double aortic arch, right aortic arch types I and II

WEGENER'S GRANULOMATOSIS - include also bronchocentric granulomatosis, Churg and Strauss or other granulomatosis, hypersensitivity angiitis of Zeek, lymphomatoid granulomatosis, midline lethal granuloma

General References

The following books and articles provided invaluable source material in the preparation of this book. Their excellent tables and lists formed a nucleus for many of the gamuts.

Burgener FA, Kormano M: Differential Diagnosis in Conventional Radiology. (ed 2) New York: Thieme Medical Publ, 1991

Chen JTT: Essentials of Cardiac Roentgenology. Boston: Little, Brown, 1987

Edwards JE, Carey LS, Neufeld HN: Congenital Heart Disease. Philadelphia: W.B. Saunders, 1965

Eisenberg RL: Clinical Imaging: An Atlas of Differential Diagnosis. (ed 2) Rockville, MD: Aspen Publ, 1992

Elliott LP: Cardiac Imaging in Infants, Children, and Adults. Philadelphia: Lippincott, 1991

Felson B: Chest Roentgenology. Philadelphia:W.B. Saunders, 1973

Felson B (ed): Dwarfs and other little people. Semin Roentgenol 1973;8:260

Felson B (ed): Congenital heart disease. Semin Roentgenol 1985;20:110, 220

Fraser RG, Paré JAP, Paré PD, Fraser RS, Genereux GP: Diagnosis of Diseases of the Chest. (ed 3) Philadelphia: W.B. Saunders, 1988

Fraser RG, Paré JAP, Paré PD, Fraser RS: Differential Diagnosis of Diseases of the Chest. Philadelphia: W.B. Saunders, 1991

Gedgaudas E, Moller JH, Castaneda-Zuniga WR, Amplatz K: Cardiovascular Radiology. Philadelphia: W.B. Saunders, 1985

Grainger RG, Allison DJ: Diagnostic Radiology. (ed 2) Edinburgh: Churchill Livingstone, 1992

Heitzman ER: The Lung: Radiologic-Pathologic Correlations. (ed 2) St Louis: C.V. Mosby, 1984

Heitzman ER: The Mediastinum: Radiologic Correlation with Anatomy and Pathology. St Louis: C.V. Mosby, 1977

Meszaros WT: Cardiac Roentgenology. Springfield, IL: CC Thomas, 1969

Moss AJ, Adams FH, Emmanouilides GC: Heart Disease in Infants, Children and Adolescents. (ed 2) Baltimore: Williams & Wilkins, 1977

Reed JC: Chest Radiology: Plain Film Patterns and Differential Diagnoses. (ed 3) St. Louis: Mosby-Year Book, 1991

Reeder MM, Palmer PES: The Radiology of Tropical Diseases. Baltimore: Williams & Wilkins, 1981

Silverman FN (ed): Caffey's Pediatric X-ray Diagnosis: An Integrated Imaging Approach. (ed 8) Chicago: Year Book Medical Publ, 1985

Sutton D, Young JWR (eds): A Short Textbook of Clinical Imaging. London: Springer-Verlag, 1990

Swischuk LE: Differential Diagnosis in Pediatric Radiology. Baltimore: Williams & Wilkins, 1984

Swischuk LE: Imaging of the Newborn, Infant, and Young Child. (ed 3) Baltimore: Williams & Wilkins, 1989

Swischuk LE: Plain Film Interpretation in Congenital Heart Disease. (ed 2) Baltimore: Williams & Wilkins, 1979

Taybi H, Lachman RS: Radiology of Syndromes, Metabolic Disorders, and Skeletal Dysplasias. (ed 3) Chicago: Year Book Medical Publ, 1990

Teplick JG, Haskin ME: Roentgenologic Diagnosis. (ed 3) Philadelphia: W.B. Saunders, 1976

Wilson JD, et al: Harrison's Principles of Internal Medicine. (ed 12) New York: McGraw-Hill, 1991

Index